Plague, Pox and Pandemics

JACANA POCKET SERIES

The new series of Jacana pocket guides is meant for those who are looking for a brief but lively introduction to a wide range of topics of South African history, politics and biography, written by some of the leading experts in their fields.

Already published

Steve Biko
(by Lindy Wilson)
Shaka
(by Dan Wylie)
Govan Mbeki
(by Colin Bundy)
South Africa's Struggle for Human Rights
(by Saul Dubow)
Umkhonto weSizwe
(by Janet Cherry)
San Rock Art
(by J.D. Lewis-Williams)
Plague, Pox and Pandemics
(by Howard Phillips)
The ANC Youth League
(by Clive Glaser)

Forthcoming titles

South Africa at War, 1935–45
(by Bill Nasson)
Ingrid Jonker
(by Louise Viljoen)
The Idea of the ANC
(by Anthony Butler)
Walter Sisulu
(by Tom Lodge)

Plague, Pox and Pandemics

A Jacana Pocket History of Epidemics in South Africa

Howard Phillips

JACANA

First published by Jacana Media (Pty) Ltd in 2012
Second impression 2020

10 Orange Street
Sunnyside
Auckland Park 2092
South Africa
+2711 628 3200
www.jacana.co.za

ISBN 978-1-4314-0385-1

Cover design by Joey Hi-Fi
Set in Minion 10.5/15 pt
Printed and bound by ABC Press, Cape Town
Job no. 003686

See a complete list of Jacana titles at www.jacana.co.za

Contents

Acknowledgements 7
Introduction 9

1. Smallpox, 1713–1893:
'There are no people left, only stones'. 13
2. Plague, 1901–1907:
'The dreaded disorder'. 38
3. Spanish flu, 1918–1919:
'It threatens the existence of the entire race' . . . 68
4. Poliomyelitis, 1918–1963:
'The middle-class plague'. 94
5. HIV/AIDS, 1982– :
'A catastrophe in slow motion'. 111
6. Conclusion 152

Notes 155
Index 166

Acknowledgements

Both institutions and individuals have greatly facilitated the writing of this book, and to them I owe my sincere thanks.

A year's sabbatical leave from the University of Cape Town gave me the time and space to focus singlemindedly on one subject, a privilege which cannot be quantified but whose value makes it the perk of being on the academic staff of UCT. Within this generous framework I was able to work most fruitfully, tapping to good effect the resources of four institutions, UCT's Oppenheimer and Health Sciences libraries, the National Library of South Africa and the Western Cape Provincial Archives and Records Service. My gratitude goes to the staff at all of these repositories.

Fellow medical historians Anne Digby, Elizabeth van Heyningen and David Killingray, along with the staff of UCT's Centre for Infectious Disease Epidemiology Research, gave me the benefit of their knowledge and insights in commenting on specific chapters, while my friend and publisher, Russell Martin, was shrewd enough to turn my germ of an idea into this book, in the process even becoming infected himself by my fascination with epidemics.

Finally, three members of the Phillips foursome – my wife, Juelle, and our children, Laura and Jeremy – felt the secondary effects of epidemics yet again and bore these with good humour, tolerance and ready support and interest. However, they will be the first to recognise that it is unlikely that their husband/father has yet acquired immunity from further epidemic investigations.

Howard Phillips

Introduction

Epidemics – the unusually high prevalence of a lethal human disease[1] in a town, country or region – loom small in accounts of South Africa's past, almost in inverse proportion to the anxious attention they attracted while they raged. In part this is because, until quite recently, historians have not known how to incorporate them into their versions of history, dominated as they were by political, economic, social and cultural issues, from which the history of the country was constructed. In this short-sightedness, they failed to recognise that, far from existing outside these frameworks, in some separate medical paradigm, epidemics (and disease generally) are integral to every aspect of life, death and society. In the unequivocal words of a historian of global epidemics, 'Truly, an epidemic tempers a society … There is no middle ground with plague. It is the litmus test of civilizations.'[2]

It is from this holistic, social history of disease

perspective that this book proceeds, as it places epidemics firmly within the country's past and treats them as something not extraneous to the mainstream of its history. Indeed, what epidemics often do is to accentuate many features and beliefs present in society, as well as to accelerate processes already under way therein, some of which may not be easily visible to historians under normal circumstances. In this respect, quite apart from their direct impact on society, epidemics provide very revealing lenses on the past. As one historian put it graphically, they 'exposed the nerve system … of society'.[3]

The five epidemics on which this book focuses – smallpox in the 18th and 19th centuries, bubonic and pneumonic plague from 1901 to 1907, influenza in 1918–19, polio in the first half of the 20th century and HIV/AIDS since 1982 – are certainly not the only plagues which afflicted the country over the last 300 years. Another five (and more) could easily have been added: for instance, measles in Cape Town in 1807 and 1839 and in the concentration camps of the South African War, so-called Mauritian fever (probably typhus) in the Cape Peninsula in 1867–8, typhoid in Bloemfontein in 1900, typhus in the Transkei in 1917–22, 1933–5 and 1943–6, and cholera in KwaZulu-Natal, Mpumalanga and the Eastern Cape in 1980–3 and 2001–2. As for tuberculosis, its ongoing high prevalence in the country since the 1880s makes it a lethal endemic disease rather than an epidemic one.

Unlike the second five epidemics, the first five selected for investigation were particularly severe and raged beyond a single town or region, which means that they left a mark both deep and wide on the fabric of society. As the five chapters show, in a variety of ways their impact on South Africa's past was decisive. Secondly, they occurred at pivotal moments in the country's past – early in the European colonisation process, during the mineral revolution, in the midst of the South African War and World War I, as industrialisation and rapid urbanisation were getting under way, and within the eras of apartheid and post-apartheid. With all of these processes they had a two-way relationship, both affecting them and being affected by them. They thus also shed a telling light on these well-established landmarks in the country's history, but from a novel social history of disease angle. South African history should not look the same to readers after they have finished this book.

1

Smallpox, 1713–1893

'There are no people left, only stones'

> 'Wherever the European had trod, death seems to pursue the aboriginal'
>
> – Charles Darwin, *The Voyage of the Beagle*

As a natural preventive against infectious disease, isolation is beyond compare. Epidemiologists believe that until humans began to establish towns in the 'Old World' of the Middle East, Asia and the Mediterranean Basin and engage in long-distance trade, the diseases they contracted were few and far between and mainly the product of their interaction with local insects and domesticated animals. By AD 1400 such relatively healthy conditions no longer prevailed in these regions, though they still did exist in most parts of four continents, viz the Americas, Australasia and sub-Saharan Africa. Epitomising such conditions was a statement by a group of Khoekhoe leaders to the

Dutch governor of the Cape as late as 1678, that 'no particularly severe sicknesses are known among them, and Death usually contents himself with old worn out people'. To the Dutch, the Khoekhoen appeared 'generally free from … visitations [of epidemics] … a circumstance which never, or at least very seldom, happens among them, in comparison with the numbers carried off in the course of nature'.[1] However, such pathogenic innocence did not long survive the creation of Europe's commercial empires overseas from the 16th century onwards, not in the Americas, Africa or Australasia. In the pithy maxim of the author of *Ecological Imperialism: The Biological Expansion of Europe, 900–1900*, 'when isolation ceases, decimation begins'.[2]

In the zone of Africa furthest from Europe, southern Africa, the pathogenic effects of these 'virgin-soil epidemics' on the hitherto isolated Khoekhoe pastoralists of the Cape were soon felt. Without prior exposure to incoming diseases, like the Amerindians and Aborigines they lacked any acquired immunity to them. Reports of 'great sickness' among the Khoekhoen began to appear with increasing frequency in the Commander's journal from 1658, more often than not accompanied by the words 'great mortality'. In 1687, for instance, it was reported from the southern Cape that 'there is a very severe and deadly sickness among the Hottentots, who do not know what to do for it; and although they decamp and move from place to place, the sickness still pursues them … The burning fever drags many, both old and young to their graves.'[3] That earlier in the month an 'infectious fever' with similar symptoms had been raging in Cape Town, causing many deaths, suggests the source from which that disease reached the southern Cape.

Under the weight of these recurring pathogenic blows and the ongoing erosion of their economic, social and political structures by Dutch colonisation, Khoekhoe autonomy and stability became increasingly compromised and fragile. What tipped the society over the edge was the arrival in 1713 of what in Holland was branded 'the worst of all the harpies', smallpox.

While it existed – it was eradicated globally in 1978 – smallpox, or *Variola major*, was caused by the *variola* virus, which was easily spread from an infected person to others by coughing, talking or contact with the former's bedding or clothing. Close proximity and crowded conditions thus favoured transmission, while smallpox's high infectivity meant that any and every contact without acquired immunity to it was at risk.[4] After incubating symptomlessly in an infected person for about 12 days, the disease began to make itself felt by a rising fever, a splitting headache and then its tell-tale symptoms, blisters in the throat and a rash that quickly ripened into blisters on the skin, which turned into pus-filled pustules particularly on the face and limbs.

In 20 to 30 per cent of cases death followed within 7 to 10 days; recovery in those who did not succumb took 5 to 6 weeks, during which time the patient remained infectious. By surviving the disease, such people acquired lifelong immunity from it, but often at high personal cost. Many were left grossly scarred by pockmarks, blind and infertile. Tellingly, the 19th-century Zulu term for smallpox was *ingqakagqa*, meaning 'the face is spoilt', while British soldiers were sometimes referred to in Xhosa as *amarwexu* ('people who have the mark of smallpox'). In many societies around the world such facial disfigurement was enough to cause depression, self-concealment and even suicide. For the disease itself there never was an effective remedy; the best that biomedicine could offer by way of treatment was comprehensive and supportive nursing.

Yet, humans did contrive two preventive measures against smallpox, both, unwittingly, based on the principle of immune response. In China, the Middle East and perhaps parts of Africa, already before 1550 healers were taking pus or scabs from a smallpox victim and introducing this into an uninfected recipient's system by insufflation or inoculation[5] to yield a milder version of the disease: this induced immunity in a person, provided he or she survived. In the 18th century the immunity-by-inoculation technique, or variolation, was taken up in elite circles in Europe whence it spread to its colonies.

The second preventive measure, devised by the English country doctor Edward Jenner in the 1790s, drew on the technique of inoculation but instead used fluid from pustules produced by cowpox, an unpleasant but benign disease caused by a virus closely related to *variola.* This procedure, known as vaccination, conferred immunity far more safely, thereby sidelining inoculation and revolutionising prevention of the disease around the world in the course of the 19th century. With justice, the *Encyclopedia Britannica* calls it 'one of the great discoveries in the history of medical science'. So significant a watershed in the prevention of smallpox was vaccination that what follows will examine the smallpox epidemics which afflicted southern Africa from the 18th century in two distinct epochs, that before and that since the invention of vaccination.

The pre-vaccination age

Three times in the pre-vaccination era, in 1713, 1755 and 1767, smallpox struck the subcontinent via Cape Town. On all three occasions it arrived from Dutch colonies across the Indian Ocean (twice Batavia and once Ceylon) where it had flared up at regular intervals since 1602 as part of an ongoing global pandemic in the early modern world. On all three occasions the vector seems to have been smallpox-infected clothing belonging to passengers or crew who developed the disease during the ten-week-long voyage to the Cape. Twice, in 1713 and 1767, the first cases occurred among laundrywomen who had washed these clothes; in 1755 the first victims were probably second-hand clothes dealers who had traded them. As in Boston, Buenos Aires, Bahia and London, other smallpox-smitten seaports of this era, Cape Town's periodic epidemics owed much to the recurring presence of a significant number of non-immune people there, especially children. As a recent historian of the disease explains, this non-immune population 'grew back steadily after each outbreak, like underbrush after a wildfire … But when the susceptible population had built up to a critical level the balance would tip in favour of smallpox and the arrival of just one or two infected cases could trigger a devastating outbreak.'[6]

With so vulnerable a population present in Cape Town, cases multiplied rapidly once smallpox struck. Mortality was at the upper end of the range, especially among the town's children and the whole region's Khoekhoen. For example, in 1713, 25 per cent of

Dutch colonists, 35 per cent of the Dutch East India Company's slaves and an even higher percentage of Khoekhoen died in the space of six months. 'Where before one saw youths amusing themselves [in the streets] it now became deathly, and one scarcely saw a house that was not closed by death or sickness,' observed a contemporary gloomily,[7] while another was told that Khoekhoen 'died as if by hundreds, so that they lay everywhere along the roads as if massacred as they fled inland with kraals, huts, and cattle'.[8] Confirming this decimation, early in 1714 a handful of Khoekhoen arrived at the Castle from the Piketberg area, requesting that the Commander appoint new captains for them to replace the four who had died of smallpox. They reported that 'scarcely one out of ten members of their society had survived'.[9]

In 1755 and 1767 the mortality rate among colonists and slaves was lower – perhaps as a result of immunity acquired and the arrival of new, already immune immigrants – but among the hyper-vulnerable, children and rural Khoekhoen, the disease's impact remained dire. Empty kraals, unattended cattle and Khoekhoe burial mounds heaped with stones bore silent testimony to the lethal nature of the disease well beyond Cape Town.

As with the earlier epidemic, the 1755 and 1767 outbreaks penetrated deep into the interior too,

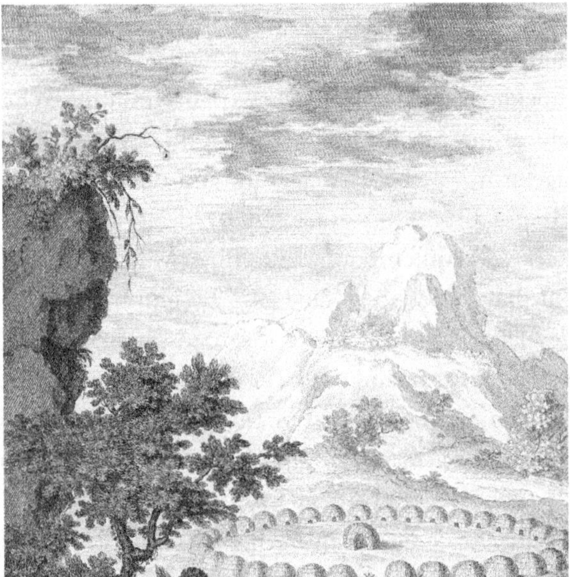

A Khoekhoe burial early in the 18th century, based on a description by a VOC official who witnessed the smallpox epidemic of 1713. Such funeral rituals would have been common early in the epidemic, before it assumed cataclysmic proportions among the Khoekhoen. (From Peter Kolbe's The Present State of the Cape of Good Hope *in NLSA Iconographic Collection, ARB 8495)*

to Namaqualand and the Transgariep in the north and also to the Overberg and the Transkei in the east. Indeed, so unprecedented was the scale of the decimation it caused among the Xhosa in the Transkei that, to prevent the disease infecting others, their traditional mode of caring for the sick in their huts was abandoned and, instead, those with smallpox were sent into the bush to die in isolation. Their relatives had to be ritually purified before being allowed back into the fold. Among them, as among all communities ravaged by smallpox in the subcontinent, 'the very name of this disease had ever since been sufficient to make an African tremble', as an explorer a generation later discovered.[10]

The response of the Dutch East India Company (VOC) authorities to the three epidemics matured markedly over the course of 54 years, in keeping with growing medical knowledge and administrative capacity. Thus, the lack of an organised medical and administrative response in 1713, when every household had to fend for itself, stands in striking contrast to Governor Tulbagh's panoply of countermeasures in 1755 and 1767, which were drawn up with the assistance of Cape Town's doctors. They aimed, in the first instance, at keeping at bay still infectious carriers of smallpox aboard arriving ships through tighter medical inspection and, if need be, quarantine.

If these failed and the disease nevertheless came ashore, a second set of measures sought to curb its spread and, with the aid of the Dutch Reformed Church, to provide nursing care for the sick in two isolation houses, one for indigent colonists and one for slaves. These measures clearly perceived the town's slaves as the likeliest portal of infection, for they flagged their places of accommodation and work for special monitoring, especially if these involved washing laundry, baking or butchering meat. The latter two trades were singled out because contemporary medical opinion believed that fresh meat and newly baked bread readily attracted 'all foul humours' in the air.

This medical opinion was, however, clearly less taken with the latest biomedical innovation against smallpox, inoculation, for, although this had been introduced to Holland in 1748 and although Governor Tulbagh had been sent a pamphlet outlining its ability to prevent a recurrence of the 'immense destruction' of 1755, it was never adopted by the VOC administration at the Cape. Why not is puzzling, since inoculation was practised elsewhere in the Company's domains, while it is not unlikely that some Asian-born slaves in the Slave Lodge bore the mark of having been inoculated as children and could demonstrate its benefit when an epidemic raged around them. Perhaps the answer lies in the conservatism of both the town's doctors and its burghers. The latter 'were not yet become rational enough to adopt inoculation', commented a visiting doctor dismissively in the 1770s.[11] Yet such blanket scorn may be excessive, for there is some evidence to suggest that inoculation may have been practised privately, but on a very limited scale.[12]

If conservative biomedicine alone shaped the VOC's preventive measures, in the realm of individual treatment it was not by itself, for it had to share this market with European folk remedies, traditional Khoekhoe and African healing systems, and the hybrid medical practices brought from the East by slaves. Against smallpox, however, whatever these had to offer – bleeding, balm, buchu or a brew of lemon water and herbs – was equally ineffectual. This meant that, to the bulk of the population, it was religious belief that offered the surest support amidst an epidemic.

Slaves who had practised Islam before their enslavement in the East would have put their faith in *azeemats*, or talismans, containing Quranic quotations, which they would have worn if permitted to do so; Calvinist Christians fasted and prayed to God to stay 'His smiting hand' from meting out 'our well-deserved punishment',[13] while both Khoekhoen and Xhosa cast around, as was their wont in the face of evil, for the malevolent human source of such an extraordinary calamity. To many Khoekhoen, it seems, the answer was obvious, for they were heard 'cursing the Dutch who they said had bewitched them'.[14]

Not that they were alone in pointing fingers. As already indicated, the sanitary gods (operating through Cape Town's doctors) quickly fingered slaves as likely carriers of infection, and to these they subsequently added the town's Khoekhoe female domestic workers, for inspections at the height of the 1755 epidemic had revealed that they were living in crowded, fetid and unhygienic conditions from which 'inevitably an even greater disaster must arise'.[15] They were therefore ordered to leave these dwellings at once for the homes of their employers. Those who did not were forced to move into the countryside to work on farms.

The channelling of such women to farms points to a significant economic consequence of the epidemics in the Western Cape, a shortage of labour. To offset the loss of many of their slaves and seasonal farmhands to smallpox, farmers energetically recruited new labourers from among the now immune Khoekhoe survivors, probably because slaves had become too expensive to buy on account of their shortage. In the south-western Cape many remnants of shattered Khoekhoe families had thus become permanent agricultural workers by 1720, while in the Overberg this took until the 1770s. The epidemics of 1755 and 1767 were therefore 'major catalysts in the Overberg Khoikhoi's transformation into farm labourers', concludes a recent account. 'Khoi kraals ... became reservoirs of farm labour to trekboer farmers in the vicinity.'[16]

Every sector of already eroding Khoekhoe life was assailed by the three smallpox epidemics of the 18th century. Flight from its ravages left their traditional grazing land open to occupation by colonists; vacated huts were torched in their absence to root out possible infection; leaders who had given their social and political structures cohesiveness and direction died, covered in grotesque pustules; and, most destructively of all, their numbers were thinned suddenly, critically and irreparably by a disease which, along with others, whipsawed through their ranks repeatedly, not only killing by the score – including successive generations of children – but also leaving many of those who survived disfigured, physically and psychologically wrecked, and sterile. The consequent low birth and high child mortality rates would have produced among the Khoekhoen, just as they did among the indigenous population of Hawaii a century later, an 'unwavering downward trajectory of the population'.[17]

Whereas the settler population was able to rebound from its severe losses in the same three epidemics because of the arrival of immigrants from Europe (most of whom were young, with an acquired immunity to smallpox), there was no source of demographic renewal for the Khoekhoen. Scattered on farms throughout the Cape, their language, history and culture a fading memory, they were transformed from independent, pastoral Khoekhoen into servile, colonial Hottentots. Like the Arawacks, the Aztecs and the Aborigines, their traumatised society and its structures collapsed under the sustained pressure of colonisation and contagion. Any post-mortem of this process must allocate to the *variola* virus a decisive role.

The vaccination age

Just as the spread of the *variola* virus worldwide from the 16th century and the dissemination of inoculation through Europe and its colonies in the 18th century exemplify the early phase of globalisation, so does the diffusion of vaccination from 1798 mark an acceleration in this process. Within 18 months of the publication of Jenner's path-breaking work, news of it had reached Cape Town, and by 1803 vaccination was tentatively being rolled out by the authorities, to a combination of euphoria and disbelief among the residents that a disease so deadly to the town for three generations – they have 'a horror [of it] beyond all belief', observed a visitor[18] – could so easily be prevented by little more than a pinprick. By 1805 over 5000 vaccinations had been performed in the town, while an expedition into the western Karoo had been undertaken to spread the gospel of vaccination inland. A new age in the history of smallpox in southern Africa was dawning.

The proof of the vaccine was in the preventing, and this was soon demonstrated during outbreaks of the disease in Cape Town in 1807 and 1812. In neither did the mortality rate top 1 per cent of the population. Compared to the 25 to 35 per cent in the 18th century, this must have seemed well-nigh miraculous. The Governor declared that this confirmed 'in the most convincing manner' the efficacy of vaccination, which the new British rulers had strongly pressed on Capetonians. At the height of the 1812 epidemic, for instance, a team of doctors had systematically vaccinated the town's fearful inhabitants street by street. A father 'had the satisfaction of seeing that, from out of the arms of my second daughter, then about four years old, whom I held on my lap during the operation, not less than one hundred and eighty individuals were vaccinated'.[19]

Not that all Capetonians readily opened their arms to this newfangled preventive procedure or any of the other counter-measures so energetically undertaken by the British administration, whether in the form of closures, fumigation, flagging infected dwellings and contacts, or quarantining. Religious principles, cultural traditions, fear of the unfamiliar – it will be remembered that vaccination's predecessor, inoculation, was virtually unknown at the Cape – aversion to being vaccinated arm-to-arm with an animal disease, suspicion of innovations by the alien British administration and tales about the noxious effects of vaccination, all fuelled avoidance. Christians and Muslims of such a mind thus shunned or hid from vaccinators. Some Muslims were even reported to have sucked the 'poison' from the arms of newly vaccinated co-religionists. Therefore, as the epidemics of 1807 and 1812 faded from memory, the government's zeal to vaccinate the population ebbed, so that, within a generation, vaccination had become 'all but unknown among the greater body of the people'.[20]

As the number of non-immune Capetonians began to rise in this way again, so did smallpox recur in epidemic form there, thrice more in the 19th century, in 1840, 1858 and 1882–3.

In 1840, as in 1812, it arrived aboard a slave ship on its way from Mozambique to Brazil, while in 1882 it was brought to Cape Town on a steamer from Britain. Given that the slaver was a prize ship captured in 1840 by the Royal Navy's Anti-Slavery Squadron, it is apparent that the pathways of smallpox to Cape Town in the 19th century had changed from the Asian origins of those of the 18th century, reflecting the shift in the Cape's position from the Dutch to the British maritime network after 1806.

Britain's growing military, commercial and transport footprint in southern Africa also meant that the 19th-century epidemics were not slow to move beyond the Cape Peninsula. That of 1840 swiftly spread to the Transkei, while that of 1858 travelled beyond the Orange River, at least as far as Lake Ngami and the Limpopo River. Smallpox 'always comes from the *south*', an explorer was told by the Ngwato.[21]

Several other outbreaks occurred deep in the interior too, north of the Orange River in 1803–4 and again in the early 1830s, in the Ciskei in 1856–7, in Colesberg in 1866, in Kimberley in 1883–4 and in Johannesburg in 1893. Since these were not obviously linked to outbreaks in Cape Town, it may be that other pathways of infection were opening up, perhaps by human movement overland from Mozambique as the subcontinent was drawn into wider economic networks and the beginning of the mineral revolution.

Although in absolute terms the three 19th-century epidemics which hit Cape Town claimed many more victims than their 18th-century predecessors,[22] relative to the town's far larger population in the 19th century, their toll was appreciably lighter – respectively 12 per cent (1840), 8 per cent (1858) and 7 per cent (1882–3) of the population. This was primarily due to the revival of official vaccination campaigns after their lapse between 1812 and 1840 – 'How's your poor arm?'

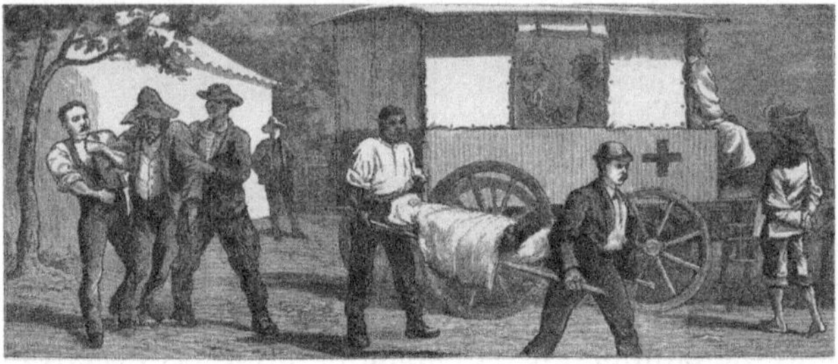

Smallpox in Cape Town in 1882. Stricken locals are being brought to the special smallpox hospital at Rentzkie's farm near present-day Brooklyn. (The Graphic, *13 January 1883)*

became a common greeting among townsfolk in the 1870s[23] – and the imposition of stricter and more thoroughgoing steps to curb the spread of smallpox once it had broken out. Influenced by the public health movement then emerging in Britain, these added the clean-up of insanitary conditions and the systematic, district-by-district provision of medical and material relief to the poor to already well-established counter-measures like special smallpox hospitals, quarantine, isolation, disinfection and the burning of victims' clothes and bedding.

As in 1812 too, these did not go uncontested, especially by Muslim Capetonians, whose sense of identity and political voice had begun to blossom with the end of slavery in 1838. Still trusting in *azeemats* and traditional spiritual medicine, they objected with increasing ardour to biomedical preventives like vaccination, isolation and fumigation, arguing that these ran counter to divine will, while the special smallpox hospitals they rejected for not providing *halaal* food or facilities for performing the necessary rituals on the dead prescribed by Islam. They suspected that the staff there were all too ready to bury Muslims as they did non-Muslims, i.e. in a hurry and in a coffin. Malays 'despise all our nostrums, and look with contempt on all prophylactics', complained one local doctor.[24]

As in countless other instances in Asia, Europe and the Americas, where burgeoning biomedical precepts and institutions collided with traditional beliefs and practices, epidemics brought out this clash of cultures very starkly. While in 1840 and 1858 imams denied the prevalence of smallpox in their community and turned a blind eye to the concealment of new cases in a bid to stave off official intervention, by 1882 Muslims' resistance had swelled to include threats to sanitary inspectors searching for new cases and even holding a public protest meeting at which a community leader warned that he would shoot anyone who tried to remove his children to the smallpox isolation hospital. To a councillor who insisted that the law was superior to religion, he replied, 'No, I beg your pardon.'[25] Recognising that discretion was the better part of valour when dealing with enfranchised voters at election time, the town council thereupon arranged for *halaal* meat to be supplied to the hospital, for a Muslim nurse to be employed to help tend patients in a dedicated Muslim ward, and for a tent to be erected for ritual washing of the Muslim dead.

Such official compromises were not favoured by many of the town's whites, however. To them, Muslims' intransigence during the epidemics confirmed the stigmatised stereotype of them which they had long held: that they were 'other', antediluvian and anti-modern in outlook and practice, and hidebound by traditionalism. 'The Malay doctrine of predestination tends to make them reckless in such matters, no precautions, in their opinion, having any effect in averting what is decreed,' snorted the *Cape Times*.[26]

Not that holding a non-biomedical view of disease was the only reason to oppose public health measures against it. In Kimberley in 1883–4 several leading doctors with links to the diamond-mining industry publicly denied the presence of smallpox among migrant workers, instead diagnosing them as suffering from a rare skin disease. They appear to have done so lest admitting that the dreaded smallpox was raging would have affected the supply of labour and materiel, thereby interrupting mining operations. Led by Cecil Rhodes's bosom friend Dr Leander Starr Jameson, the anti-smallpox doctors waged a fierce war of words against their smallpox-averring fellow-doctors for over a year. Consequently, measures to curb the epidemic were sporadic or, in the mining compounds, nonexistent, and cases topped 2000, with mortality at 3.5 per cent of the population. Only when the colonial government eventually called in a string of outside doctors to diagnose the disease – the last declared that it was smallpox 'pure and simple' – was the cover-up terminated and vaccination, fumigation and isolation vigorously pursued. The conspiracy of denial, by retarding action and sowing doubt about the need to be vaccinated, had been responsible for no small percentage of the 700 deaths in the town. It was one of the 'most diabolical uses to which the medical profession was put for the sake of the mining interest', concluded one historian.[27]

Blaming a malevolent individual or group for a catastrophe like an epidemic was as usual in the 19th century as it had been in the 18th. In Cape Town, a belief that what appeared to be contrary conduct by Muslims was partly driven by an animus against white citizens yielded rumours that the former were deliberately seeking to infect whites with smallpox, by carrying their dead on biers through the streets in a 'reeking procession' or by rubbing shoulders with them in public spaces or even by getting Muslim laundrywomen to drape whites' washing over smallpox corpses before returning it to its owners. As with most finger-pointing during crises, such accusations reveal more about the accuser's state of mind than the accused's deeds. But such thoughts sometimes led to action. At least twice, whites were so inflamed by these tales that they attacked Muslim residents with carbolic acid to punish them for spreading the disease.

Not that white Capetonians had a monopoly over conspiracy theories to explain smallpox epidemics. Others were regularly held responsible for such evils too, whether it was Basters accusing Korana of bringing the disease to them in 1804, Hurutshe Tswana blaming Ndebele in 1835 for ignoring ancestors' instructions and so provoking an epidemic, or Transkei Xhosa seeing the British colonial government's hand in a disease which was 'secretly destroying them' in 1842.[28] It has even been suggested that rumours that the British were introducing smallpox into Xhosaland in 1856 helped fuel the sense of being under siege that led to the desperate millenarian Cattle Killing there in 1856–7.[29]

For the devotees of universal religions, however, there could be only one source: smallpox was indubitably an instrument of divine action. To Muslims, the *takdier* of Allah ('will of God') behind this was unknowable but might perhaps be assuaged by an appeal for mercy through fasting and prayer. For Christians, the epidemic was a divine punishment for sin, verily 'a remarkable visitation of God … [which] spared neither old nor young, but swept them away as with the besom of destruction', as one missionary put it powerfully in 1815. The only escape lay in repentance and prayer, prompting many to mend their ways and return 'to their bibles and to their knees before God'.[30] Indeed, some were so struck by the magnitude of the scourge that they saw in it a herald of deeper things afoot, the coming of the Millennium.

In the shorter term, it was in the field of public health that the smallpox epidemics of the Victorian era had the most reforming impact. Not that this was swift to occur or comprehensive in scope, for, as with most epidemics, little of the flurry of street-cleaning and sanitary improvement which they triggered long survived their passing. Rather, it was their periodic returns that reminded authorities of unfulfilled agendas. Thus, it took two smallpox epidemics and 28 years for the Cape Town municipality to act on the issue of overfull cemeteries first raised in 1858, while it took the colonial government 16 years to enact legislation (in 1856) giving them the power to take extraordinary action against outbreaks of infectious disease, and then another 27 years and two epidemics to plug some of its biggest gaps.

In like fashion, it required the spur of the 1882–3 epidemic to persuade them to collect and publish reports on the state of health in the Cape Colony annually, for Cape Town finally to appoint a municipal medical officer of health and a sanitary engineer (both firsts in southern Africa), for the villages adjoining it to amalgamate into a single municipality possessing the financial muscle to tackle the primitive sanitary conditions there, and for Kimberley to have a Board of Health created to assume responsibility for the health of its residents.

Even with these structures in place, the public health reforms that followed in Cape Town were slow to come and limited in their scope: the closure of the town's crowded and unhygienic old cemeteries in 1886 (not without forceful opposition from the Muslim community), the construction of municipal wash-houses in 1888 and the removal of the insalubrious shambles on the shore of Table Bay to a distant location in 1889. Even the hostile calls in the Cape Town press after the 1882–3 epidemic for the residential segregation of Muslims and 'other uncleanly natives'[31] on account of their disease-inducing and -disseminating lifestyle – 'the sooner the Malays are made to reside in a separate district the better for all concern[ed]', ran one[32] – were not acted on until 1901 and the outbreak of another epidemic, this time of bubonic plague.

For two centuries smallpox was to southern Africa what the plague had been to medieval Europe in terms of its devastating demographic destruction and the terror it evoked. An old San hunter remarked graphically that where it walked, 'there are no people left, only stones'.[33]

Yet, the invention of vaccination as an effective preventive against it gives it another significance in southern Africa's history too, for, as this prophylactic measure was disseminated through the region in the 19th century by medics, missionaries and ministers, its success gave to it and to the biomedicine which it represented *par excellence* a powerful boost as that medical system sought to penetrate the wider population. Indeed, it would not be far off the mark to suggest that the spread of biomedicine in the 19th century was led by the tip of a vaccinating lancet.

2

Plague, 1901–1907

'The dreaded disorder'

> 'In most communities the mere mention of plague breaking out with such dramatic suddenness would have a disastrous effect on the public mind'
>
> – *Rand Daily Mail*, 22 March 1904

If the movement of human beings was central to the spread of smallpox, the mobility of this species was of only secondary importance in the first epidemic to strike the subcontinent in the 20th century, plague. This is because plague is primarily a disease of rodents, caused by the bacillus *Yersinia pestis*, which is most commonly spread from an infected to an uninfected rodent by fleas. Only if infected rodents die in an epizootic in such numbers as to deprive the now infected fleas of rodent hosts, do they seek out other mammals in the vicinity to bite in search of blood, thereby infecting them too.

If these mammals are of the human variety, the effects of such a bite are swift and often lethal, for humans are particularly vulnerable to *Yersinia pestis*. Within three to six days, generalised symptoms like a raised temperature, splitting headache, inflamed eyes and giddiness appear, soon followed by the tell-tale sign of bubonic plague (the commonest form of the disease), the appearance of buboes, or inflammatory swellings in the groin or armpits. On average, 60 per cent of those so infected die within a week of the emergence of buboes.

In bubonic plague, therefore, it is the movement not of humans but of rodents and their fleas that is central to the spread of the disease. The movement of humans becomes significant only in cases of bubonic plague in which *Yersinia pestis* so grossly infects patients' lungs that it can be spread from person to person by coughing. In such circumstances it turns into airborne pneumonic plague, spreading from human to human with such alacrity and virulence that death occurs before buboes even appear. Pneumonic plague is usually even more lethal than flea-borne bubonic plague, claiming 70 to 90 per cent of cases.

It seems likely that twice before the 19th century the die-off of rodents in this cycle reached such levels that their fleas turned to humans, producing two great pandemics, the so-called Plague of Justinian of the 6th century AD and the grim Black Death of the 14th century. The latter, along with one of its later derivatives, the Great Plague of London of 1664–5, caused such mortality that these two outbreaks were indelibly and gruesomely impressed on the European mind for generations to come, making the name of the disease, plague, a synonym for 'epidemic'. Plague thus possesses the 'richest genealogy of fear in the Western psyche', notes one of its historians.[1]

There is no evidence that southern Africa was touched by either of these pandemics, probably because it was isolated from their centres in Asia, the Middle East, North Africa and Europe. However, by the end of the 19th century this was no longer the case, thanks to the expansion of global trade during the intervening centuries and the consequent incorporation of the subcontinent into the international maritime network. Thus, when, between 1894 and 1896, bubonic plague broke out in a number of Chinese and Indian ports, and from there began to spread swiftly across the seas aboard steamships carrying grain, alarm bells began ringing in southern Africa as loudly as on other continents at the possible approach of what has been labelled the third plague pandemic in world history.

Alerted by horrifying reports of thousands of plague deaths in Asia and anticipating that it was unlikely that the 'Oriental' plague (as it was pejoratively dubbed by contemporaries in the West) could be kept at bay forever, governments in southern Africa anxiously readied themselves against the arrival of what one local doctor called 'the dreaded disorder'.[2] The discovery of a suspicious case in Lourenço Marques in Mozambique in January 1899 quickly prompted an inter-state conference on plague control to be held in Pretoria, attended by representatives of the Cape, Natal, the Transvaal, the Orange Free State and Mozambique. Drawing on the recommendations of the 1897 International Sanitary Conference in Venice, they drafted guidelines according to which any outbreak should be met. Nor did this remain armchair planning for long. Even as they debated, a suspected case of plague was reported from Middelburg in the Transvaal, sending a *frisson* of dread around the room and triggering a plague scare across the region. The Transvaal instantly imposed restrictions on the movement of Indians – the Middelburg suspect was a recent arrival from India – while authorities in the Cape and Natal sought to tighten port health controls. Initially these appear to have worked, for no further cases were reported that year, while early in 1900 a Mauritian visitor diagnosed with plague in Durban was immediately isolated and a ship arriving in Cape Town with a dead captain and sick crewmen was promptly quarantined by a vigilant port health officer and its entire cargo of grain burnt. When these precautions failed, it seems to have been primarily because they were overridden by Britain's military authorities.

In October 1899 southern Africa descended into a three-year war between Britain and the Boer republics of the Transvaal and the Orange Free State. Certainly, this swelled the number of humans on the move as a vastly expanded imperial army conducted its military operations across all four territories and refugees from the Witwatersrand crammed into Cape Town, Port Elizabeth, East London and Durban. More important as far as bubonic plague was concerned was the imperial army's spiralling need for fodder for its horses. This it sourced from all over the globe, most conveniently from Argentina, where cases of plague had begun to appear in September 1899 in the grain-exporting port of Rosario, though it was some months before this was officially confirmed.

From Rosario to Cape Town it is not difficult to discern a hay-strewn trail, and from this to identify the first of the ports of significant entry of plague into southern Africa. Signs of a large die-off of rats in a section of Cape Town harbour restricted to military use (which included the offloading and stacking of forage) began to appear in September 1900. 'The stench was unendurable, and ... they had had to have the floors up to remove the dead rats,' reported an ordnance officer.

'He himself had seen numbers of sick rats coming out to the open in daylight, in a dazed state so that you could catch them with your hand.'[3] However, news of this ominous epizootic among harbour rats was not conveyed to Cape Town's medical authorities by the local military command.

Indeed, it was not until February 1901, after two civilians working in the military section of the harbour had fallen ill and been diagnosed with bubonic plague, that the city's medical officer of health learnt that 'the dreaded bubonic plague – the scourge of India – had at length made its appearance in our midst'.[4] By the middle of March over 130 cases of plague had occurred in the Peninsula, 56 of them fatal.

Although it was most probably via cargo on ships from Cape Town that the colony's second port, Port Elizabeth, was infected soon thereafter, it is worth noting that, despite the substantial increase in the amount of fodder being transported into the interior, plague rarely spread far inland from these ports. This may have had something to do with the low winter temperatures in the interior, which made rat fleas less active. Thus, it was only in the immediate hinterland of these ports that cases of plague were reported in 1901–2, and even then in very small numbers.

If Cape Town was the first point of significant entry for bubonic plague from abroad, then Durban was probably the second, though on a smaller scale. In November 1902 its harbour was infected by rats in a shipload of lucerne hay from Argentina. Within days the disease had spread inland as far as Pietermaritzburg.

The district surgeon of East London claimed that it was from Durban too that his town was infected, probably arriving by sea early in 1903 in a cargo of rat-infested grain. From there, its passage into the Border region during the ensuing weeks can be systematically tracked by noting outbreaks among either rats or people along the railway line northwards, for instance at King William's Town, Kei Road, Queenstown and Seymour.

Circumstantial evidence also suggests that it was from East London that the one serious penetration of the deep interior by *Yersinia pestis* emanated early in 1904, when a young Indian labourer, in the throes of developing pneumonic plague, arrived in Johannesburg from the coast and proceeded to infect his family and their neighbours in that city's tightly packed Coolie Location. He had gone to his brother's house there 'sick with fever' to try to recover from the disease overtaking him.[5]

That, in the few instances that the disease did reach far inland, it was most probably in this pneumonic form suggests that neither the rat hosts of *Yersinia pestis* nor its flea vectors were good or rapid travellers across land, especially during the winter months. The result was that, as elsewhere in the world, the plague was most serious at points where it first came ashore, viz the heart of seaports, where it raged briefly and intensely but never comprehensively.[6] Even in Cape Town, the worst-hit port in Africa, its incidence was under half a per cent of the population.

Out of all proportion to these figures was the dread that plague evoked. Apart from the tales of the Black Death and the Great Plague of London, what prompted such fear was the disease's lethality once contracted. Here, Cape Town's case mortality rate (the percentage of cases dying of the disease) of 48 per cent presents a frighteningly different picture of the disease from its incidence, while those of Johannesburg (73 per cent) and Durban (72 per cent), where pneumonic plague dominated, were quite terrifying. The message was clear: if a person contracted the disease, he or she was likely to die.

The trajectory of plague outbreaks was thus usually a sudden, sharp onset, generating a great deal of trepidation and panic as deaths rapidly mounted, but then followed by a levelling-off of cases and a steady abatement of the disease, punctuated by sporadic flare-ups. In Cape Town, for instance, the outbreak was clearly waning by early in May 1901, ten weeks after its onset, while in Durban its incidence began to fall progressively after three months. In Johannesburg, with its explosive pneumonic start which claimed 55 lives in the first week, the epidemic tapered off inside a month.

By the end of 1907 even the occasional flare-ups among humans had ceased, and *Yersinia pestis* in southern Africa was henceforth largely confined to its natural host, rodents, among which it became endemic for the first time in the region's history. For animals of the order *Rodentia* this was a legacy of no little import, just as it was for the handful of humans who were to be bitten by their infected fleas – sometimes fatally – over the next decades.

Medical authorities at the beginning of the 20th century understandably believed that the measures which they had taken in response to the epidemic had been instrumental in curbing it, and it is likely that they were – at least in part – correct. However, if this was so, it was not because their measures were based on a complete understanding of the disease. At the time, biomedicine's knowledge of plague – as of all infectious and contagious diseases – was in the throes of a watershed transition as a result of the germ revolution of the late 19th century. That plague was caused by *Yersinia pestis* was generally accepted, but exactly how it was transmitted was not clear. That rats were somehow involved was recognised, if only

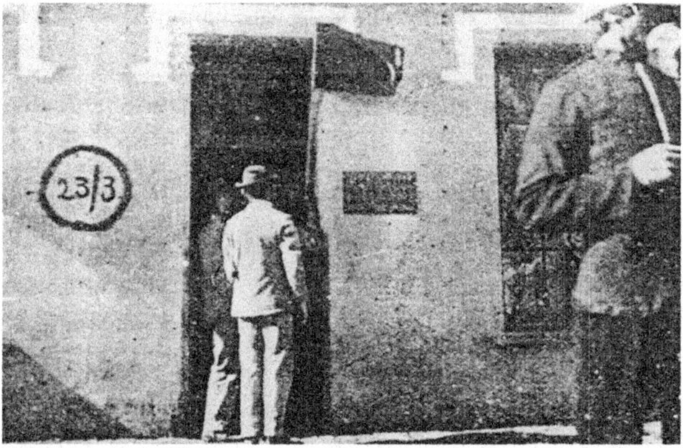

A house in Cape Town in which a case of bubonic plague had been found on 23 March 1901. The house is about to be shut up by officials who have marked it with the date (23 March) and a yellow flag next to the door. A policeman with a truncheon stands on guard in front of the house. (Cape Argus Weekly Edition, *3 April 1901)*

because their habitat and behaviour so obviously fitted in with prevailing sanitary ideas that dirt meant disease. But where the pathogen came from – the filth-saturated soil, overcrowded and insanitary dwellings, or the rat itself – and how it was transmitted – directly from the rat, from one person to another, or even, as one bacteriologist claimed, from the rat via its fleas – was still under intense debate.[7]

Thus, it was possible for one old-school doctor in Johannesburg to blame the epidemic on the 'accumulation of filthy matter [which had] imparted to the ground a surface of poisonous excrescence, which … [was] transformed into a deadly vapour which impregnates the atmosphere',[8] while at the same time a British adviser on plague to the Cape government could maintain that rats and mice became infected by eating contaminated food 'or by passing over infected clothing or places' and then 'convey[ing] infection to healthy houses'. According to him, 'Filth associated with darkness and dampness is peculiarly favourable to the growth of the microbe, whereas cleanliness, sunlight, air and dryness are its most deadly enemies, and destroy it almost at once. Old, dilapidated, dark, insanitary, and overcrowded houses, premises, and localities infected by rats are particularly dangerous.'[9]

Whether the disease could pass from person to person was another bone of medical contention, with most doctors convinced that it was highly infectious, hence requiring cases and contacts to be tightly quarantined, while a few argued that it was not and that, consequently, 'the segregation of contacts – i.e., persons who have been living or in communication with plague patients – is useless as a preventive, and should not be attempted'.[10] One senior medical officer even went so far as to pooh-pooh the priority given to sanitary and quarantine measures, insisting that 'only the well recognised but quite unexplained periodicity of Plague outbreaks, whereby they come to a conclusion in some six months ... could be relied upon to terminate its course'.[11]

This diversity of medical opinion was reflected

in the steps taken to combat the plague epidemic in southern Africa as health authorities sought to cover all their bases by recommending an all-encompassing, blunderbuss approach, though often with a particular emphasis, depending on how up-to-date their medical officers were. Almost all took sanitarianism as their point of departure, making those living under insanitary conditions their first target, especially if they were not white-skinned, as the wielders of political power were.

Then, as now, the acute threat to life posed by an epidemic readily called forth existing social prejudices to find a scapegoat. Given the increasingly racialised nature of local society, the 'others' at whom whites invariably pointed their fingers were Africans and Indians living in 'their' towns. Such racial stigmatisation saw the former as out of place in the city and as 'mere visitors to the town', as Natal's Secretary for Native Affairs expressed it.[12] In Cape Town, the city's medical officer of health believed that 'uncontrolled Kafir hordes were at the root of the aggravation of Capetown slumdom brought to light when the plague broke out. [Because of them] it was absolutely impossible to keep the slums of the city in satisfactory condition.'[13] In like fashion, in King William's Town the acting resident magistrate spoke for many local whites when he insisted that it was Africans 'with their filthy habits, who brought the disease into the town', even though it was clear that it had arrived with rats aboard a train from East London;[14] while in Durban similar racialised tunnel vision saw alarmed whites clamour for action against 'the public health menace' posed by the city's Africans, despite the fact that the plague outbreak stemmed from the harbour where rat-infested grain had been landed from Argentina.[15] In Port Elizabeth, the district surgeon's prejudices against those who were not white-skinned went even wider as he imputed the plague outbreak to the 'mixed population in Port Elizabeth – Hottentots, Kafirs, Chinese, Indians – [who] specially predispose to overcrowding, and insanitary dwellings'.[16]

On the other hand, in Johannesburg it was the Indian residents of Coolie Location, the centre of the outbreak there, who attracted whites' sharpest condemnation for what the *Rand Daily Mail* and many of its readers perceived to be 'filthy habits and gross perversion of the most elementary sanitary rules ... Under any circumstances, he [the Indian] makes filth, and surrounds his habitation with the germs of every disease under the sun ... Keep those coolies as far away as possible from the centres of [white] population,' it urged. About Africans living in Coolie Location similar sentiments were expressed.[17]

Given the fear let loose by the arrival of plague,

it comes as no surprise that such crude racial pathologising informed almost every official measure taken against it at the behest of the special plague committees or boards set up to direct or advise on these steps. It provided them with a compelling justification for forcefully tackling both the immediate epidemic enemy and a host of other apparently related social ills once and for all, amounting to the pursuit of what the historian Maynard Swanson has memorably (if a little obscurely) labelled the 'sanitation syndrome', which he defined as a 'societal metaphor … [which] powerfully interacted with … racial attitudes to influence the policies and shape the institutions of segregation'.[18] 'Epidemic expediency' (or 'an epidemic of expediency') may be both more accurate and more telling a phrase.

In Cape Town, Port Elizabeth, Durban, King William's Town and Johannesburg, the main urban centres hit by the plague, steps against the epidemic therefore began with house-to-house searches for new cases and contacts, which concentrated on areas where Africans and Indians dwelt. On top of everything else, both groups were also accused of concealing these cases as long as possible out of benightedness (so the authorities claimed) or mistrust of the plague officials' inspections (so residents explained). Certainly, on several occasions in Cape Town, families refused to allow plague cases or their contacts to be removed to the special plague hospital or the nearby quarantine camp, and the police had to be called in. Flight by contacts so as to avoid quarantine was also not uncommon.

In Johannesburg, quarantining went even further, for its new, British-dominated municipality was determined to show that, unlike its Boer predecessor, it could deal with a crisis swiftly and efficiently. Within hours of the disease, which was rampant in Coolie Location in March 1904, being officially diagnosed as pneumonic plague, the entire location had been cordoned off by the police and no one was allowed to leave or enter it. 'In view of the possibly widespread affection [*sic*],' explained the Rand Plague Committee's medical officer, 'it was deemed wiser to treat all the inhabitants, for the time at least, as suspects and not as mere contacts; it would have been impossible to have inspected them daily had the cordon been broken and the inhabitants allowed to go where they pleased.'[19]

Dwellings in which cases were discovered were usually also dealt with in a racially selective way, stemming from existing prejudices linking race to insanitary living conditions. In Port Elizabeth, Durban and King William's Town such buildings occupied by Africans or Indians were commonly demolished or burnt and their inhabitants sent to an emergency tent camp. However, if the inhabitants were white or

Coloured, the building was fumigated and disinfected and the erstwhile residents allowed to return to it after the epidemic had passed. Cape Town scapegoated Africans even more precisely, out of a combination of racial prejudice, fear, paternalism and the fact that so many of the early cases there were discovered among African labourers living in slum areas like District Six. Whether plague cases had occurred where they lived or not, in terms of the epidemic provisions of the Public Health Act some 6000 of the city's Africans were forced to leave their homes and were escorted by soldiers to a tent camp at Uitvlugt Forest Station on the Cape Flats, five miles from the city centre. There they were all meant to be medically examined, inoculated and housed in supposedly more sanitary accommodation. Coloured and white Capetonians were removed to a different emergency camp if their homes were infected but allowed to return once the buildings had been disinfected and fumigated.

Johannesburg once more exceeded its fellow cities in its sanitary zeal. The Rand Plague Committee there had all of the 3178 people it had corralled at Coolie Location – 1612 Indians, 1420 Africans and 146 Coloureds – removed under armed guard and sent to a municipal farm at Klipspruit, twelve miles west of Johannesburg, where they were put into tents and huts in two racially separate isolation camps a mile apart, both surrounded by a contingent of troops. Only clothing, bedding and utensils which had been disinfected were allowed into the camps; all other possessions – save laundry belonging to white customers – had to be left behind for fumigation or burning. Back in Johannesburg, the empty Coolie Location was then burnt to the ground by, paradoxically, the Johannesburg Fire Department as the soil was deemed too contaminated and the buildings too insanitary to be renovated. A spectator of this fire, the young M.K. Gandhi, noted perceptively that the torching of Coolie Location was 'essentially a theatrical display', calculated to reassure white Johannesburg that no stone would be left unturned to safeguard their health.[20]

Racially selective measures were in evidence too in the restrictions placed on travel by rail or sea out of infected areas by Indians or Africans. Such would-be travellers had to have a plague pass first, and this required a prior medical examination to ensure that they were showing no signs of the disease. Yet, even possession of such a pass was no guarantee of freedom to travel, as several Africans found when they arrived at a station, only to be turned back by guards deployed there specifically to prevent Africans who did not look well from embarking or disembarking. In the event, these barriers were often avoided by Africans, who opted to go to smaller stations where there were no guards. Reflecting on this experience of discrimination, the Xhosa-language newspaper *Imvo Zabantsundu* regretted that 'regulations for public safety could not be carried out without causing grievance among Natives' and urged that 'if the laws are to be administered in this land of mixed populations it will be well to apply them with due regard to common sense'.[21]

Such common sense was certainly not in evidence when Port Elizabeth's Plague Board sought to compel local Africans to be inoculated with Haffkine's brand-new anti-plague vaccine in 1901.[22] To achieve this, it insisted that plague passes would be issued to Africans only if they had already been medically examined and inoculated. Coming on top of other instances of discrimination against them, this requirement that they alone should be subjected to an unknown vaccine was the last straw, triggering an unprecedented general strike by African workers in the city. Whites 'may travel wherever they desire without restrictions of this sort – why, then, not the Natives?' demanded one of their leaders angrily.[23] The withdrawal of their labour in the midst of the war, especially that of stevedores, was enough to convince the Board of the unwisdom of its decision and it relented, issuing a new proclamation which, at least on paper, made the prerequisites for travel applicable to all residents of Port Elizabeth, irrespective of skin colour.

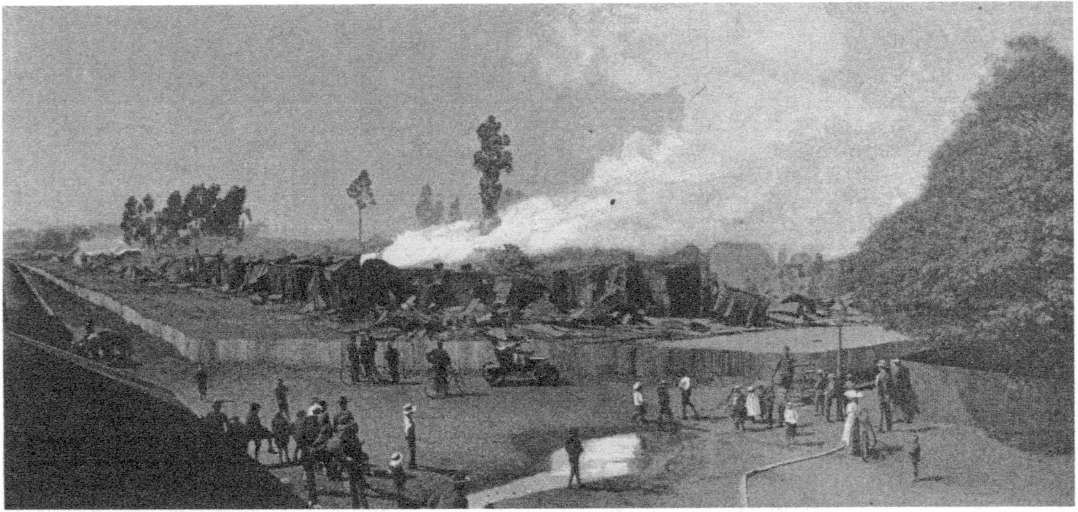

Coolie Location in Johannesburg goes up in flames on 8 April 1904 in a bid to purge the site of pneumonic plague and allow it to be redeveloped for the expansion of municipal services. (The Graphic, *4 June 1904)*

Elsewhere in southern Africa local circumstances dictated the authorities' stance on inoculation. In Cape Town the colonial medical officer of health had already decided that, except among the virtually captive Africans at Uitvlugt, mass inoculation with this novel vaccine would not be pushed too strongly, especially in view of its often unpleasant after-effects, the deaths of several of those inoculated (including two nurses at the plague hospital) and popular rumours among the underclasses that inoculation was sinister in intent and aimed to spread the plague among them, not prevent it. For similar reasons, authorities in Durban and Johannesburg also soft-pedalled inoculation. As the Rand Plague Committee's medical officer patronisingly put it, 'The native is a particularly nervous person when he is subjected to unknown forms of treatment, and it was very advisable to avoid any form of scare.'[24]

However, in King William's Town, learning very smartly from 'the deplorable results which have followed the stupid bungling of the matter at Port Elizabeth',[25] the equivalent authorities went out of their way to win the confidence of the town's Africans over inoculation by first consulting them about it at a mass meeting and then making it optional for all races. The response was in telling contrast to the fiasco in Port Elizabeth a month before: some 20,000 King William's Towners inoculated free of charge.

Probably the only anti-plague measure on which all humans in southern Africa were at one was the need to kill rats. In every town, even the threat of an outbreak was enough to persuade local authorities to step up their standard rat-catching campaigns, but now followed by bacteriological examination of the dead rats for evidence of *Yersinia pestis*. If an outbreak did subsequently occur, the campaign was accelerated, reaching frenetic levels. Extra teams of rat-catchers were hired, the public was offered a bounty of 3d for every rat brought to a municipal depot, and sales of rat-traps, rat-poison and rat-proofing soared. Every plague report of this period breathes this anti-rat fervour – for instance, the district surgeon of King William's Town reported with satisfaction in 1903 that 'a war of extermination was waged against rats, many thousands being destroyed'.[26] In all, probably over a quarter of a million rats were killed during southern Africa's plague years. Paradoxically, epidemiologists nowadays hold that, in the midst of a plague epidemic, the killing of rats causes their infected fleas to desperately seek out other mammals on which (or on whom, if they are humans) to feed, thereby spreading the disease more widely.

Compared to these rat deaths, the number of humans who died of plague of one form or another in the subcontinent between 1901 and 1907 was small, viz 958, a mere fraction of the deaths from this disease in Asia during the epidemic there.[27] Though the case mortality in southern Africa (55.9 per cent) was on a par with the high figure elsewhere, the small absolute number of deaths does raise the question of the overall significance of this epidemic for the region. Certainly, the health officer for Natal, Dr Ernest Hill, rated it as of little importance. He declared that he had 'studiously avoided' the word 'epidemic' in his *Report on the Plague in Natal* 'as conferring too much importance on any outbreak which in seven months attacked no more than about three and one-third per thousand of the entire population in Durban, being a far less prevalence than that of Enteric Fever or Dysentery among the European portion'.[28]

Nor, in sheer demographic terms, was Hill wrong. But a historical approach must go beyond this to the disease's lasting social and political import too, in particular to its role in shifting the residential segregation of Africans in towns and cities across the subcontinent onto a new plane. As Swanson argues, 'It was the merest step of logic to proceed from the isolation of plague victims to the creation of a permanent location for the black labouring class … With the plague emergency the definitive step of quarantine and segregation was taken.'[29]

In Cape Town, the emergency camp at Uitvlugt

to which the bulk of the city's Africans had been dispatched in the midst of the plague crisis was, in 1902, turned into a permanent location for them called Ndabeni. This was made possible only by the passage of special legislation to bar them from living elsewhere in the Peninsula, which superseded the Public Health Act provisions under which they had been forcibly removed and constrained there for over a year. Africans' attempts to challenge this compulsory resettlement by open protest, a rent and train boycott, and through the courts had proved in vain in the face of official determination to corral them in a single location where their comings and goings could be controlled by the authorities. Their leader's pointed question 'By what legal process or right of law or equity have you … acted?' was ignored, as was his poignant reminder that 'Natives are sensitive human beings and therefore capable of feeling as well as [a] white man of any grade. Let us assume a *vice versa* position and what would the white man feel and say?'[30]

Quite simply, the outbreak of plague had provided an unchallengeable opportunity, in the face of a terrifying threat to life, for segregation lobbyists within the white establishment to push aside opposition to their long-sought goal and effect a mass removal of Africans to a single, controllable location on the outskirts of the city, something they had been punting publicly since at least 1899. In this regard, one of their strongest supporters, the *Cape Argus*, felt that the plague might be 'a blessing in disguise' for Cape Town.[31] In the words of the historian of this removal, 'The plague emergency … was the precipitant cause of the government's decision to bring a location into being almost overnight. But had the various governmental authorities been readier to decide who should act, and possessed the legal authority to compel Africans to live in a location, it might well have been created before the plague struck the city.'[32]

In Port Elizabeth the plague epidemic performed a not dissimilar function, giving the white powers-that-be a powerful argument to attain – at least in part – a goal for which they had been striving since the mid-1890s, viz the closure of four haphazardly run African locations in the inner city and the transfer of their inhabitants to a single, well-ordered and well-controlled location on the edge of the town. Step 1 in this direction was quickly taken at the behest of the Plague Board, amidst the panic sparked by the plague's arrival. This was the removal of the residents of infected houses in these locations and their demolition, even though a site for a new location to accommodate those evicted had not yet been secured. Step 2, the identification of all remaining insanitary dwellings in the inner-city locations, their condemnation as unfit for human habitation and the eviction of their residents, followed within months, despite the new location, called rather optimistically New Brighton, still not being ready. By the time that it finally was, in May 1903, the African population in the inner-city locations had already been more than halved by evictions and flight. Those evicted had moved to a tent camp provided by the town council, were sharing accommodation with location residents whose dwellings had not yet been destroyed or were renting cheap rooms somewhere in the city or in the shantytown rapidly mushrooming beyond the municipal boundary at Korsten.

The opening of the custom-built location at New Brighton, five miles from central Port Elizabeth – 'a grand native town that … would furnish a model for other towns and districts throughout South Africa', as the *Eastern Province Herald* ambitiously boasted[33] – was intended by the authorities to be the culmination of their plan for the mass removal of Africans. To this end, in mid-1903 they formally disestablished what was left of three of the four inner-city locations, razed them to the ground and evicted their remaining inhabitants, confident that they would now stream to New Brighton. But in fact most preferred to go to Korsten, which was much nearer to the city centre and not subject to the restrictive regulations in force at New Brighton. Try as the authorities might over the next two years to convince, cajole and coerce Korsten's Africans to move to New Brighton, they met with little success. 'Everybody knew that New Brighton was a white elephant, and the government wanted to blacken it with natives,' quipped a local newspaper.[34] Not until special legislation was passed in 1905, making Africans living five miles beyond the municipal boundary (as at Korsten) subject to eviction too, did numbers at New Brighton begin to rise steadily. As the historian of that location remarks, it had taken just four years from the Plague Board's first steps in 1901 to accomplish 'what the Port Elizabeth town council had been attempting to achieve for the past forty years: to force many African residents in the inner locations out of town'.[35]

In King William's Town the mere possibility of plague spreading there in 1901 was enough to spur the town council into creating a new location on the edge of the town. It hoped that this Ginsberg Location would become a magnet for Africans residing in the town, to whose presence white townsfolk had been objecting since at least 1898. When the plague did actually break out there in 1903 and again in 1905, efforts were renewed to induce the town's Africans to move to the new location, but in vain. It was not until 1907, after a third plague outbreak, that the town council finally abandoned persuasion for legal sanction, invoking provisions under the recent Municipal Act of 1906 to 'require all Natives, with certain stringent exceptions, to live in the locations'.[36]

In Durban, the colonial government's long-cherished wish to do the same with regard to Indians and Africans was also rekindled by the plague's arrival. Natal's Department of Public Health wanted 'All coloured people of the working class whose services after sundown are not indispensable … [to] live in their own locations … [so that the] haunts of the labouring class would then be known – confined to the place of work and the legitimate place of residence.'[37] Consequently, a Native Location Act was passed in 1904, but when it came to implementing it the municipality jibbed at the cost of establishing a location and so postponed action indefinitely.

As might be expected, Johannesburg was at the other end of the spectrum when it came to determination to entrench racially based residential segregation at any cost. Having hastily removed the Indian and African inhabitants of Coolie Location to Klipspruit when the plague struck, its British-dominated town council sought to take advantage of this situation to recast the city's racial geography permanently into a clearly segregated colonial city from which the old, loosely segregated city-centre locations had been removed and in which racially mixed areas were a thing of the past. There should be 'a proper, whole-hearted treatment of this coloured question' which would unscramble the way in which 'the Malays, Indians and Kaffirs were jumbled all over the place' under overcrowded and insanitary conditions, maintained the chairman of the municipality's Public Health Committee.[38] 'The wholesale removal of the natives from the town would place us in a better position to protect ourselves against the outbreaks of disease and would lessen their frequency and virulence,' agreed *The Star*.[39]

In pursuit of this vision of a modern, orderly and sorted British colonial city, the town council invoked a recent by-law to compel all the city's Africans not residing on their employers' premises to move to Klipspruit by 1 April 1906 to join those Africans already dumped there in 1904 from Coolie Location. A petition against this forced move by 275 African residents of the Kaffir Location close to the city centre – 'as it was not our desire nor wish to go to Klipspruit', which was far away and could only be reached by train[40] – received a polite but unaccommodating response from the council. To the council's regret, such unilateral action against the Indian community was not possible lest the Government of India object, and so those at the Indian plague camp at Klipspruit were reluctantly allowed to filter back into Johannesburg.

This ad hoc manner in which Klipspruit became

an African location belies its lasting historical significance. Despite its distance from Johannesburg, its proximity to a sewage farm and its generally insalubrious living conditions, it became a prime focus of residence for Johannesburg's African population because of the space to expand which its environs offered. In 1934 it was renamed Pimville and, as such, became the nucleus around which subsequent townships were constructed after World War II to accommodate the thousands of Africans flocking to the City of Gold. In 1963 these 26 townships, housing close to half a million Africans, were bracketed together under the name Soweto, at the heart of which lay the original Klipspruit Location, dating back to the hurried removal in 1904 in the shadow of the plague epidemic. From small germs do mighty townships grow.

It is in this episode that the larger, long-term impact of *Yersinia pestis* on southern Africa is visible. Even before its constituent territories were unified into a single state in 1910, its policy-makers were responding to the growing African presence in its towns and cities in ways not dissimilar. Ndabeni, New Brighton, Ginsberg and Klipspruit bear testimony to this fact. The epidemic expediency provided by the plague accelerated existing social and political trends significantly in favour of single, segregated state-run locations situated at a distance from city centres. In terms of where they were located, how they were run and the degree of control over the residents which they afforded, they marked a significant break with both the racially mixed, inner-city districts and the loose urban locations where most Africans had lived in the subcontinent's towns until then. In shifting the organisation of communities away from this casual, flexible and informal situation, *Yersinia pestis* had an impact out of all proportion to the number of lives it took. This many-times magnified effect derived from the frightening connotations which the word 'plague' had for contemporaries steeped in Western culture and the greater authority attached to biomedical opinion by policy-makers because of the germ revolution. Paradoxically, in the case of the plague epidemic of 1901–7 in southern Africa, neither was justified.

3

Spanish flu, 1918–1919

'It threatens the existence of the entire race'

Three hundred thousand (or 6 per cent of the population) dead in six weeks; tens of thousands of wives and husbands turned into widows or widowers virtually overnight; hundreds of thousands of orphans created at a stroke. These stark statistics sum up the grim impact of the devastating epidemic of so-called Spanish flu,[1] which raged through South Africa in October–November 1918 and again, less virulently, in August 1919. Short, sharp and savage, 'Black October' (as contemporaries called it) became a synonym for the country's worst epidemic ever, for it outdid in intensity, range and lethality every other epidemic in the subcontinent before or since.

This vicious epidemic was part of a global pandemic of highly infectious influenza which swept around the planet in 1918–19 in three waves. The first and last of these were widespread but not unduly serious, confining most of those it struck to bed, but no more.

The second wave was quite the opposite in character, for it rapidly assumed a deadly form, claiming one victim after another.

First noticed in military training camps in the United States early in 1918, the pandemic was spread from there by land and sea, primarily by the mass movement of troops and sailors to and from the main theatres of World War I. In this way the tail-end of the mild first wave reached Durban early in September 1918, carried there by soldiers returning from campaigns in the Middle East and German East Africa. From Durban it spread into the interior of Natal and then to the Witwatersrand, where it prostrated thousands of miners but caused relatively few deaths. It would only 'produce temporary inconvenience without serious loss', forecast the local Reuters correspondent confidently, and 'in view of the fact that such a very large number of people have been affected, the fact that there has been only one death must be considered to be reassuring'.[2]

But even as these optimistic words were being written, the deadly second wave of the pandemic was starting to penetrate the country from a different direction. Having arrived in Cape Town aboard two troopships in mid-September, it raced inland as the now demobilised men from these ships returned home by train. In even as remote a spot as Tsolo in the Transkei, within days of a batch of Native Labour Corps soldiers disembarking from the troop train from Cape Town, 'sickness has become rife amongst both races in village and country', reported the local magistrate, 'and people are being brought in to [the] local doctor by wagon and sledge loads'.[3]

By mid-October, almost the entire country had been overwhelmed by the same plight, as demobilised soldiers and migrant workers fleeing home from infected cities and mines spread the disease far and wide. Nor was it any longer just laying people up in droves, but it was also killing a frightening number of them. In Cape Town, deaths topped 400 per day, 40 times greater than the usual daily toll, while, at the height of the epidemic in Kimberley, it was estimated that if deaths were to continue at the current rate, the entire population of that city would be wiped out in 16 months. In Bloemfontein, shops, offices and workshops were closed for want of staff, public transport and services like the post office were paralysed, and ailing residents were dropping dead in the streets. 'All this week the hand of the disease has lain heavily on the town,' observed a weekly newspaper, 'and so uncanny was the stillness in the streets and shops that we might have been in a city of the dead.'[4]

As eerie was the silence in the countryside. 'For two weeks a great solemn hush has prevailed,' wrote a correspondent from the Cathcart district in the Eastern Cape. 'No one is to be seen, no one to be heard; no life on the farms, no work in the lands. Lord influenza and his followers have held the countryside in their grip.'[5] Corpses lay alongside the sick in kraals, animals wandered in the fields unherded, and cows went unmilked. The epidemic 'threatens the existence of the entire race', concluded a resident of the Transkei fearfully.

As in most epidemics when life is under dire threat, blame-mongering soon began along the many fault lines of South African society. Thus, some whites blamed Africans for recklessly spreading the disease as they fled from epidemic hotspots – there were even calls for them to be barred from the trains to curb this – while some Africans blamed whites and their government who, they believed, wished to kill them. For instance, white relief workers in the Ciskei reported that they were preceded by a local 'telling the people that this disease was a device of the Europeans to finish off the Native races of South Africa, and as it had not been quite successful, they were sending out men with poison to complete the work of extermination'.[6] For many rural Africans, therefore, hospitals and whites offering medicine or anti-flu vaccine were to be shunned at all costs. 'The people simply w[oul]d not have us,' noted an Anglican bishop trying to help treat

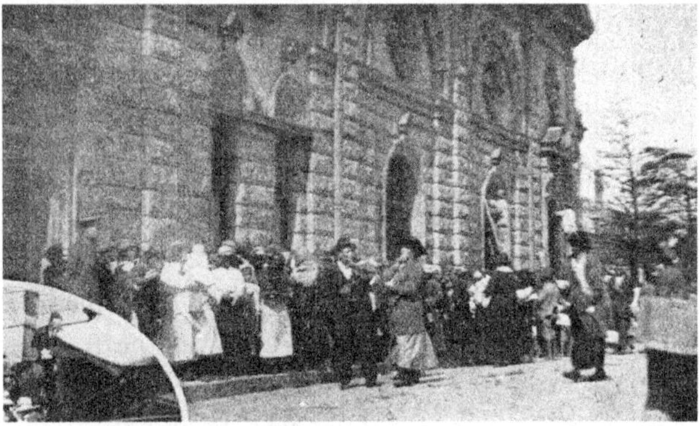

'Black October' 1918 at its height in Cape Town.
Above: *An all-race queue, consisting mainly of women, outside the City Hall, waiting to collect food, soup and a bottle of hastily mixed anti-flu medicine.*
Below: *A young woman who had collapsed in the street outside the City Hall is helped into an ambulance.*
*(*Stage, Cinema and S.A. Pictorial, *9 November 1918)*

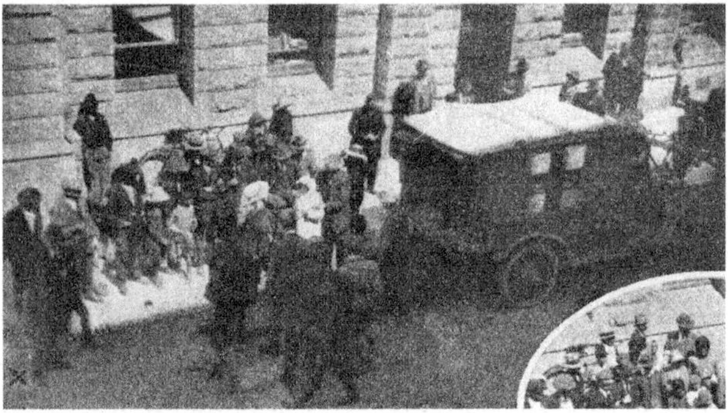

Africans in the Transkei. 'One stood outside his hut & insisted his child was better: another woman took our medicines but said we had come to poison them.'[7]

Given that it was wartime, not a few patriotic fingers were pointed at Germany and particularly at its use of poison gas. A Bloemfontein newspaper reported that it had received numerous letters concerning 'the Kaiser's alleged share in or authorship of this calamity',[8] while one doctor insisted that 'Spanish influenza is not a suitable name. German plague is more accurate.'[9] Local white politics delivered up its own brand of accusations too. Several diehard members of General Hertzog's National Party believed that General Botha's government had deliberately let the flu loose to wipe out his political opponents, while others expressed the view that the epidemic was a divine warning that 'we should not interfere in wars which did not concern us'.[10]

Fuelling the panic and terror behind such accusations was a rising tide of corpses. Residents of the country's towns and cities were hardest pressed to cope with this. In Cape Town municipal carts toured the streets, picking up those who had died at the roadside, while families resorted to all manner of transport to convey their loved ones to the cemetery – private cars, taxis, trollies and even wheelbarrows. The office of the Cemetery Board was besieged by crowds wanting to arrange burials, while morgue attendants, undertakers and clergymen were swept off their feet by the immense demands placed on them. An Anglican minister was put on permanent standby at the city's main cemetery, while the Mayor's chaplain went there every day to officiate at any funerals for which there was no minister available.

In Kimberley, funerals went on into the night by the light of car headlamps. Coffins were in short supply, making it necessary for some of the dead to be buried wrapped only in a blanket. Many of these corpses were placed in mass graves, a measure to which the giant De Beers mining company also turned on its own property when the soaring number of its dead African miners made continued use of the Kimberley location's graveyard impossible. In this cemetery itself, recalled an officiating clergyman, African flu victims were buried in a fresh mass grave every day between 2 and 4 pm, irrespective of their religion: '25 bodies were placed in it, each in a blanket. Then we sang, I said prayers, and then a thin layer of soil was thrown over them. Then came the next 25 bodies. Usually 100 bodies were buried in this way every day ... but sometimes it was 125 and once 150. That required 6 consecutive services.'[11]

Clearly, the influenza that scythed through the population with such deadly effect was not ordinary seasonal flu. The H1N1 flu virus that caused it was a wholly new strain of the disease, to which no one in the world had prior immunity. Like ordinary flu, it was spread by coughing and sneezing and so was transmitted most effectively in crowded spaces; but, unlike ordinary flu, it rapidly penetrated deep into an infected person's lungs rather than lodging in the upper respiratory tract as most flu viruses do. Therein lay the source of its particular virulence, for its fulminating presence deep in the lungs laid the way open for viral or bacterial pneumonia, which were the chief killers in 1918–19. Laboured breathing, a high fever, crackling sounds from the lungs, bleeding from the nose or mouth, and a dark tingeing of the skin were frightening, tell-tale symptoms, along with a very distinct odour, like very musty straw, 'so pungent', recalled a survivor, 'it just came into your nostrils with a bang'.[12]

Developing primary viral pneumonia usually meant death in three days – hence the colloquial label *driedagsiekte* – but in that pre-antibiotic age secondary bacterial pneumonia often produced the same result, though not as swiftly. In many young adults with a strong immune system, infection triggered an immune over-response (known as a cytokine storm) so massive that it, in effect, caused acute respiratory disease syndrome and death. This may explain the high mortality among those in the 18–40 age-group, a very distinctive feature of the Spanish flu around the globe. The fact that this group also contained the bulk of the workforce probably contributed to the disproportionately high toll among them, for, as breadwinners, many continued to go to work instead of staying in bed and being nursed, which was probably the most effective treatment available at the time.

For doctors were at a loss to know how to treat the disease. 'We had a rough idea that care was necessary, that fresh air was an essential,' admitted one, 'but as to medical treatment our minds were fogged.'[13] Thus, the medicines they recommended ranged from aspirin, quinine, Epsom salts, phenol and cinnamon tablets to hastily concocted special flu mixtures and vaccine. All were equally useless. Poignantly, the son of a Cape Town doctor recalled his father's reaction when a newly married couple he had been treating for Spanish flu died within days of each other: 'It was then I first saw my father cry,' he recounted. 'He was sobbing in sorrow and in frustration at his impotence.'[14]

Nor were practitioners of medical systems other than biomedicine any more successful in their treatment, though this did not stop the quacks among them from making grand claims to the contrary or commercial opportunists from exploiting the situation. For instance, Commando Brandy was advertised as being sure proof against 'Huns or Flu', while Sibbalene antiseptic skin ointment applied to the inside of the nostrils was touted as a guarantee against infection.

In the end, in the absence of any sure cure, most South Africans probably put their faith in folk remedies, patent medicines and time-honoured nostrums and practices like fleeing to a remote area or self-imposed isolation. Many Africans turned to a traditional herbalist, *sangoma* or *isanuse* (witch-finder) to check the disease. As a result, smelling out by witch-finders of those deemed responsible for the extraordinary wave of deaths increased sharply, as did attacks on those identified as witches or wizards – so much so, in fact, that in 1919 the Transkeian Penal Code was amended to lay down stiffer penalties for witch-finding.

Of course, given the commitment of the new South African state to biomedicine, this brand of doctoring alone enjoyed official support. Thus, the medical assistance it did provide was exclusively biomedical in nature. For instance, the central government's fledgling, three-man sub-department of public health circulated to the public the latest medical advice from Britain on how to treat epidemic influenza, advertised for doctors and nurses locally to send to districts where these were in particularly short supply, and pressed state laboratories to develop an ad hoc anti-flu vaccine in double-quick time. But these measures were not co-ordinated and were as effective as trying to fight a veld-fire with an armful of watering-cans.

Given the sub-department's serious organisational and staffing deficiencies, the best co-ordinated official action to combat the epidemic was taken by municipal authorities around the country. With the assistance of thousands of public-spirited volunteers eager to do their bit during the war, they set up temporary hospitals, opened relief depots to supply soup, food and medicine to badly affected households, disinfected houses where cases had occurred, and conducted vigorous clean-ups of what were identified as insanitary areas. Not that the last two steps were of any actual use against influenza; they appear to have been more knee-jerk responses to the presence of an epidemic, reminiscent of steps taken in previous centuries during epidemics and intended more as evidence that authorities were indeed doing something and not just standing by as a plague claimed one victim after another.

The Union Defence Force also lent a biomedical hand once Spanish flu had waned in its camps, as many of the country's doctors and nurses were still under its control because of the war. Some of them it dispatched to specific towns and villages where their services were most desperately needed, while others were organised into three field ambulances to tour the rural Transkei and Transvaal, dispensing emergency medical care. In several places the Defence Force not only supplied medical equipment from its stores, but also admitted serious civilian cases to its military hospitals. To stricken Kimberley it sent its Acting Director of Medical Services, Colonel A.J. Orenstein, to assume control of that city's faltering efforts to stem the epidemic's tide. 'Please come at once,' the town council had begged him. 'You will be in absolute control.'[15]

With this mandate, within 24 hours Orenstein had created a comprehensive and tight-knit system which embraced all local doctors, pharmacists and hospitals and rationalised their efforts. For example, the town was divided into 12 medical districts, to each of which one doctor was assigned to deal with all calls, while pharmacists were instructed to dispense only three anti-flu mixtures; doctors had to confine their prescriptions to one of these.

Bloemfontein municipality's counter-offensive against the epidemic was equally authoritarian – 'a sort of ad hoc Soviet system', one contemporary called it[16] – only here the town's doctors dug in their heels against being assigned to one particular district. In the city's Waaihoek African township, however, 'They commandeered everything they could find,' admitted the head of the town's Central Bureau established for tackling the flu crisis, and 'if people wanted any explanation he told them to go to him later on'.[17] As far as the municipal authorities were concerned, the parlous state of the town made such high-handed direction a must. 'At no time in the history of this town has the Town Council been so absolute,' acknowledged the town clerk. 'It merely had to issue requests and vigorous workers saw to it that no one dared to refuse.'[18]

The speed and extent of the Spanish flu in South Africa – it is estimated that over 50 per cent of the population contracted the disease in the space of a month – meant that quite soon it began to wane, as the number of people with some immunity to it by virtue of having suffered a bout grew rapidly. As a doctor explained in simple terms at the time, there was 'not the same amount of fuel [left] to feed the fires'.[19]

Some 300,000 South Africans died in the six-week epidemic, i.e. about 6 per cent of the entire population, a mortality rate exceeded only in Western Samoa (25 per cent) and India (6.2 per cent). The severity of the South African experience probably owes much to the country's well-developed railway system, which facilitated the transmission of the highly infectious flu far and wide, the high number of young adult men using this system (especially migrant workers and soldiers who were returning home), and the fact that much of the population's first encounter with Spanish flu was with its deadly second wave and not its milder first wave with its immunising effect.

Of these approximately 300,000 deaths, some 78 per cent were Africans, 12 per cent Coloureds, 8 per cent whites and 2 per cent Indians. Of these, African and Coloured deaths were markedly higher than the percentage of the overall population which each racial group constituted, suggesting that, among them, living conditions were particularly conducive to the spread of the disease and that in many cases the ability to stop an infection turning fatal was seriously compromised by poor physical condition and a lack of effective nursing. As already noted, the majority of those who died were in the 18–40 age-bracket, and of these more were male than female, perhaps because in towns men were often the breadwinners who could not afford to stay at home with a touch of 'mere flu'. The only category of women of this age who were at special risk was those who were pregnant.

Geographically, Spanish flu mortality was heaviest in the western, northern and eastern Cape, the southern Orange Free State and the western and northern Transvaal. What these areas had in common was that they were on or close to railway lines stretching from those hotspots of second-wave Spanish flu, Cape Town, Kimberley, Bloemfontein and the big Karoo railway junction of De Aar. In most of

Natal, the northern Orange Free State and the southern Transvaal, Black October's toll was significantly lower. This suggests that in those parts of the country where the less virulent first wave of the disease had recently preceded the second wave, contracting a bout of the former conferred a degree of immunity against the latter. Paradoxically, therefore, the best protection against catching deadly second-wave Spanish flu was a dose of milder first-wave flu.

Nowhere is this clearer than in the adjoining rural districts of Mount Frere and Mount Ayliff in the Transkei. In the former the mortality rate almost touched 80/1000 of the population, in the latter just 14/1000. Tellingly, the nearest railway line to Mount Frere was that from the Eastern Cape and its second-wave Spanish flu, while that serving Mount Ayliff was from Natal, where the first wave of the epidemic had struck first. The same epidemic geography probably explains why young male miners at Kimberley were decimated by the second wave of the epidemic, which hit the city first, while mortality among their peers on the gold mines of Johannesburg was far lighter, as the second wave's arrival there had been preceded by an outbreak of the first wave.

Yet, the demographic impact of Black October went further than just those whom the epidemic killed. The death of pregnant mothers meant the loss of their still-to-be-born babies too – which raised knotty issues in African communities about repaying lobola if they would have been first-time mothers – while in many cases even a non-fatal bout of the disease was enough to cause a miscarriage or a spontaneous abortion. For many decades after 1918, therefore, the mark of the Spanish flu remained on South Africa's demographic structure, in the form of a reduced number of those who had been between 18 and 40 in that year and in the number of those who should have been born between October 1918 and June 1919. The latter loss explains why in 1925 the new cohort of children entering primary school was smaller than in previous years: quite simply, their numbers had been thinned by the non-birth of the usual number of children six years earlier, in 1919.

Moreover, the death of a parent, spouse or child had emotional, psychological, social and material consequences for individuals well beyond the demographic. The death of a breadwinner could produce a serious financial effect on the rest of the family, of the sort that prompted one flu widow to appeal movingly to the readers of a religious magazine. 'My dear spouse died of flu, leaving me in poverty and debt, with 5 children. Pray for acceptance and strength for me. I intend to go to the [diamond] diggings to see if I can make a living there. I will give a tithe to the Lord. Ask Him for delivery and help for me.'[20]

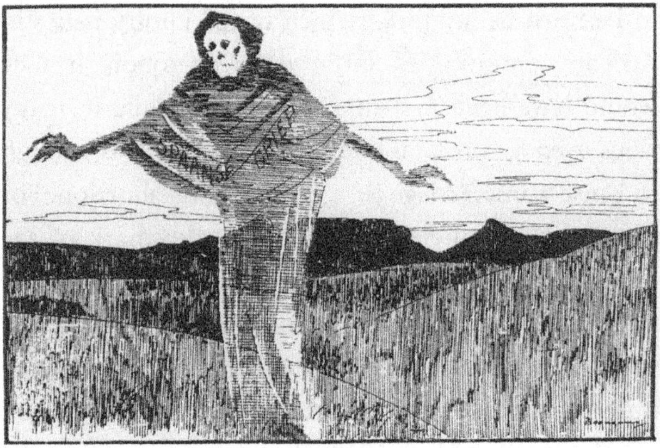

D.C. Boonzaier's chilling cartoon of the Spanish flu in Cape Town. (De Burger, *16 October 1918)*

For the hundreds of thousands of children orphaned by the epidemic, 1918 would have been at least as traumatic a year and a watershed in their lives. 'I was taken in [by relatives] as their child,' recalled one flu orphan in 1965. 'My [four] brothers and sisters were scattered. We never got together again.'[21] In most African, Indian and Coloured families such incorporation into extended families was the norm, but among whites it seems to have been far less common. Consequently, ever anxious about the future of white Afrikaners, the Dutch Reformed Church raised over £120,000 for orphanages to accommodate 'its' flu orphans. Other denominations, as well as several bodies of state employees like the police and railway staff, followed suit, some using their funds to build orphanages, others to contribute to the upkeep of flu orphans and widows in their own homes. By 1926 sixteen new orphanages had been erected and a number of existing ones enlarged, while the state had agreed to subsidise the living costs of flu orphans lodged in these institutions. In effect, the Spanish flu epidemic had transformed the provision for white orphans in South Africa out of all recognition.

Other enduring personal effects of Black October are not so easily seen by the historian. The mass grief that must have been felt by many South Africans is only hinted at by the crowds thronging the country's cemeteries all through 1919, the poignant entries in the 'In Memoriam' columns of the newspapers every succeeding October for decades, and the rise of spiritualism, of communing with the dead and of *amandiki* spirit possession in Zululand. Just how long was the emotional shadow cast by the Spanish flu is suggested by a poignant remark in 1998 by an 88-year-old man who had lost his mother in 1918. 'I still miss her', he told me sadly.

On some survivors the Spanish flu left an enduring physical and psychiatric mark too. In the 1920s numerous cases of depression, impaired heart and lung function, deafness and a susceptibility to other diseases like encephalitis lethargica, nephritis and Parkinson's disease were attributed to a bout of flu back in 1918.

Nor were many individuals' religious beliefs left unscathed by the dreadful experience of Black October. Rampant death on such an enormous, undiscriminating scale tested their faith mightily, and some found it wanting. For example, enough African adherents of traditional religion were attracted to Christianity for some missionaries to speak in public of 'the compensating blessings accompanying the ravages of the recent influenza epidemic as seen in the awakened interest among the heathen, and a desire for the Word of God'.[22] On the other hand, some African Christians were so disappointed by the inability of mainline Christianity to protect their families or comfort them in their loss that (as elsewhere in Africa) they turned their backs on the established churches and, spurred by divine visions, founded their own independent Zionist churches.

Some very devout Christians, both white and black, went even further. Interpreting the epidemic as a signal that the Millennium was in the offing, they began to preach this message and the urgent need to prepare for the Second Coming. In the environment of war, revolution, social angst and vulnerability prevailing in 1918, they attracted not a few followers, even if only temporarily.

This sense of personal vulnerability, which Black

October so intensified, also underlay record sales of life assurance in the following months, particularly as it was widely forecast that another flu wave was imminent, a possibility that the country's insurance companies did everything to highlight in their post-epidemic advertising campaigns. Thus, new life cover sold in 1919 was estimated as worth £20 million, easily a South African record in percentage terms. Insensitively, the chairman of one big insurance firm commented in his annual report, 'It is, in our opinion, all to the good that the public should have been impressed by the lesson of this severe experience to the extent of making provision as never before against the risks of death.'[23] This surge of new business allowed the insurance industry to more than recoup what it had paid out through the deaths of its policyholders during Black October.

At the public level too, the experiences of that frightful month underlined the need for action to address a host of administrative and social deficiencies which had been so starkly revealed by the epidemic. Most urgent was the need for a comprehensive system to take responsibility for the country's public health and not leave it to a heterogeneous array of local authorities of varied capacity. Three attempts to repair this omission by the makers of the Union had foundered on the rock of vested interests in the years after 1910. What Black October did was to ensure that this would not happen again. In its wake, a draft scheme to create such a system (which had been hammered out just before the Spanish flu struck South Africa) was rapidly transformed into a formal Public Health Bill, which was tabled in Parliament early in 1919. There, the prospect of a return by the epidemic drove the complex bill through all its readings with speed, yielding, at the end, the Union of South Africa's founding Public Health Act, which set up a separate, full Department of Public Health under its own minister. The government's law adviser noted that, during the debates on the bill, the experience of Black October had 'induced a spirit of compromise both in and out of Parliament, a spirit which it is doubtful would have existed except for the remembrance of what the public suffered in the epidemic'.[24]

The new Department of Public Health acted quickly to try to prevent a recurrence of Black October by requiring incoming ships fitted with wireless sets to radio to South Africa information about any outbreaks of infectious diseases on board, while all countries that had regular intercourse with the Union were requested to telegraph news of any epidemics raging within their borders. Meanwhile, all along the South African coast, port health regulations were tightened up in case the attempts to keep epidemics at bay were unsuccessful.

The elements for an early warning epidemic system thus came into being, and in 1920 these were consolidated when South Africa joined the League of Nations' International Bureau of Public Health in Paris, which issued monthly bulletins on outbreaks of epidemics globally.

If, despite these precautions, an epidemic did reach the country, the Department of Public Health sought to prepare further contingency measures too. Local authorities were prodded to draft emergency plans to deal with a recurrence of Spanish flu, while NGOs were encouraged to offer to the general public courses in basic nursing and first aid so that the country would not again be found lacking in nursing skills, as in 1918. Several Afrikaner cultural organisations and popular periodicals like *Die Huisgenoot* and *Die Boerevrouw* took this idea even further by providing elementary instruction in health to their community. 'There is not a place in our country where, in the last three months, we did not discover that we are very clumsy and ignorant in times of sickness,' noted the Afrikaner Christelike Vrouevereniging (ACVV) early in 1919. 'Now the flu has at last shaken us awake, and suddenly we recognise how ill-equipped we are in the sick-room.'[25] To redress this, it also sponsored the publication of simple medical and nursing manuals in Afrikaans, which were meant to 'contribute to making our children and ourselves healthy and strong so that we can win the battle to survive'.[26] If the *volk* were to overcome the loss of life in the South African War and now Black October, such knowledge was vital.

But even deeper socio-economic intervention was needed to deal with the wretched living conditions of so many town-dwellers, which the house-to-house visits during Black October had revealed. This was necessary not only for the sake of those residents themselves, but also to curb the risk of infection which they posed to the better-off classes. 'Germs recognize no colour bar,' a leading Cape Town churchman had warned,[27] a point taken by authorities at all levels. Building houses for their poorer residents, especially if they were white, was therefore high on the agenda of go-ahead municipalities like Cape Town and Bloemfontein already in 1919, a task made easier when the central government passed the Housing Act the following year, setting up a Central Housing Board to which local authorities could apply for funds for this purpose.

Although the housing constructed under such schemes fell far short of meeting the country's accommodation needs even for whites, it did for the first time establish the principle nationally that the central government ought to intervene in the housing market in the interests of the poor, a tenet that henceforth became a standard part of South African state policy. In the wake of Black October, even the private sector bought into this idea, albeit selectively. Led by a donation of £10,000 from its president, Richard Stuttaford, the Cape Town Chamber of Commerce piloted the construction of a healthy, uncongested garden city for middle-income Capetonians at Pinelands, while the *Cape Times* set up a fund to provide bungalows at the seaside where poor children could enjoy a holiday in a fresh, ozone-rich environment. 'Experience in the Epidemic showed what a woeful indifference to fresh air there is in the congested areas of the city,' explained the founder of what became the Cape Times Fresh Air Fund.[28]

Nor was the housing of urban Africans ignored by white authorities, though here the first priority was that such accommodation should be separate from that of whites. Thus, following in the path of Ndabeni, New Brighton, Ginsberg and Klipspruit after the bubonic/pneumonic plague epidemic of 1901–4, yet further segregated African locations were established in the years after Black October had again underlined the poor conditions under which most urban Africans dwelt. These included Langa near Cape Town, Batho near Bloemfontein and the Western Native Township near Johannesburg. The culmination of this long-developing policy towards urban Africans nationally came in 1923, with the passage of the segregatory Natives (Urban Areas) Act. As the Prime Minister, General Smuts, argued five years after Black October, 'If the principles of that Bill … were fairly applied in South Africa, we should remove what was today a grievance and a menace to health and decent living in this country.'[29] The beginning of residential segregation that *Yersinia pestis* had facilitated, the H1N1 influenza virus hastened.

In this – as in so many other epidemics in South African history – the Spanish flu had acted as an accelerator of important moves already in train in the society, like the creation of a national system of public health, the construction of hospitals, the development of popular health education, the attempt to end Poor Whiteism, the spread of Christianity and the establishment of independent Zionist churches.

But being an accelerator of the vehicle of history was not the Spanish flu's only significant role. Again, as with other epidemics, it also initiated a number of key developments in 20th-century South Africa, adding to the society major and distinctive features that were wholly novel and unanticipated, like a changed demographic structure, bereft and broken families, several hundred thousand orphans, and flu survivors physically, psychiatrically, psychologically and emotionally scarred for the rest of their lives.

In both these respects, as accelerator and initiator, the impact of the Spanish flu epidemic resembled that of another Apocalyptic Horseman, war. Or perhaps it was even more pernicious because it made no distinction between soldiers and civilians. As one flu survivor put it 60 years after Black October, 'I don't hope for anything like that flu again … That's worse than a war.'[30]

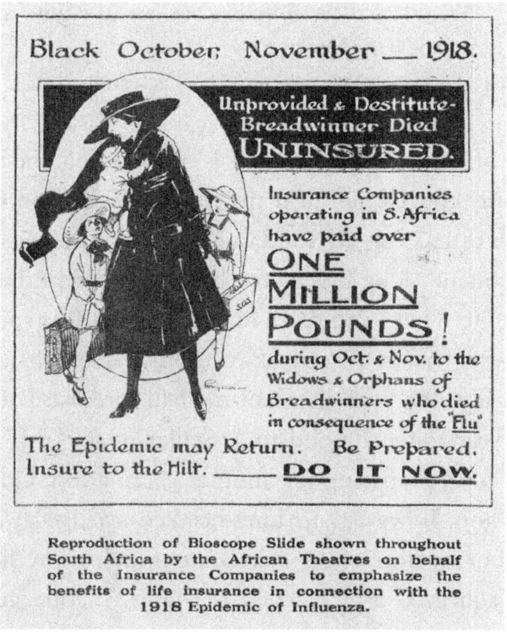

Playing on fears of a return by the Spanish flu. A cinema advertisement by the combined South African insurance industry, 1919. (Insurance, May 1919)

4

Poliomyelitis, 1918–1963

'The middle-class plague'

> 'We dreaded the summer; that was the time we knew the children were at risk'
>
> – A mother's recollection in 2002

One of my earliest memories is of being marched to a gloomy church hall near my primary school in Cape Town in 1955 or 1956 and waiting very apprehensively in a queue to be inoculated by a tall woman dressed in white. That I can recall little else about this episode suggests that it passed off without the much-feared pain that the boys ahead of me had forecast. Four or five years later, I stood in a similar queue, this time at school, preparing for another vaccination. On this occasion, however, no long-needled syringe awaited me but a white sugar-cube onto which some liquid was squeezed as I reached the table. In one gulp I swallowed it.

At the time I had no inkling that the two episodes

effectively marked the end of white South Africa's fearful 42-year encounter with what a contemporary American documentary chillingly called 'the crippler'.[1] Better known as poliomyelitis, it was, in the words of one of its South African historians, 'the number one enemy of childhood'.[2]

Infantile paralysis or poliomyelitis[3] first appeared in South Africa in epidemic form in the summer of 1917/18, some 50 years after its emergence and recognition as a distinct disease in Northern Europe and North America. In succeeding decades it returned as a countrywide epidemic to South Africa three more times, in the summers of 1944/5, 1947/8 and 1956/7, all as increasingly serious offshoots of broader global pandemics. In between, it smouldered in the background.

Unlike the great sweeping epidemics already examined, polio was not a big killer in South Africa or anywhere else. Between 1918 and 1962 it took fewer than 950 South African lives. Its significance lay in whose lives it claimed and maimed. For reasons which will be discussed later, they were disproportionately those of children of the country's small but powerful and articulate middle class, the overwhelming majority of whom were white. This class-biased incidence (which was global) makes the subtitle of this chapter, borrowed from a work on polio in Canada, equally appropriate to South Africa.[4] As a middle-class mother in Johannesburg recalled years later, 'We dreaded the summer; that was the time we knew the children were at risk.'[5]

The fear that their child might be paralysed by the disease – perhaps even killed – was more than enough to alarm every parent and so galvanise them into action. Given the social, financial, political and medical clout that they commanded, these actions produced results which gave to the fight against polio in the 1940s and 1950s an impetus out of all proportion to the risk it actually posed to the population in general. In this regard it well illustrates how a disease can be constructed as a terrifying, all-pervading epidemic at the centre of public attention when it touches those with power.

The disease with this capacity, poliomyelitis, is caused by one of three serotypes or strains of the *Poliovirus hominis.* This usually enters a person's system through the faecal-oral route, via fingers, food, water or milk which has previously come into contact with virus-contaminated sewage. The virus then incubates in the intestines for up to three weeks, 90 to 95 per cent of cases going no further owing to the body's vigorous resistance. This 'silent' form of polio produces no symptoms but leaves the people so infected unwitting vectors of the disease for up to six months, though they themselves are immune for life. If the infection does progress slightly before being overcome by the body's defences, 'abortive' polio results, producing short-lived and mild symptoms like a raised temperature, sore throat, vomiting and muscle pains. In a very small percentage of cases – especially if the infected person is physically taxed or experiencing trauma – the virus does not remain in the intestines but penetrates to the central nervous system, causing aching, debilitating but non-paralytic polio. If, however, it does not stop there but proceeds to destroy motor cells in the nervous system, the result is the much-dreaded paralysis of muscles of movement and even respiration, the latter being potentially fatal. The warning signs of this aggravation of the disease to a paralytic level are a sore neck and back and aching muscles. 'The stiff neck seemed to … spread all down my back and I felt too languid to care about anything,' recalled a resident of Bulawayo struck down in 1956. Within days, 'the paralysis had crept over most of my body, leaving me helpless … I lifted my hips – they moved only in my mind. Physically, they still clung firmly to the bed … I was as firmly embedded as a foundation stone.'[6]

In 1917/18 and again in 1944/5, it is probable that the disease assumed an epidemic character in South Africa because of the sudden arrival of one of the three strains of the poliovirus not already circulating in the country in endemic form. On both occasions the most likely vectors were South African troops returning from war-time service in the Middle East, for no sooner had they disembarked in Durban than serious cases of the disease began to appear in local battalions and among the staff of military hospitals where they were being treated. Strengthening this hypothesis is the fact that similar outbreaks were occurring at the same time in the United States, Britain, New Zealand and Australia. To each of these countries their own troops had recently been repatriated, also from the Middle East. For the later epidemics of 1947/8 and 1956/7, however, the source of the new type of poliovirus is uncertain.

Once in the country, the new strain apparently flourished best in hot but humid climatic zones, i.e. the summer rainfall areas of the then Natal and Transvaal. This may explain why the 1917/18 epidemic was largely confined to the Witwatersrand and why successor epidemics had the biggest impact there and in Durban.

Rural areas, it seems, were least affected. For example, in 1944/5 just 7 cases were reported from the entire Transkei, as against 201 in Johannesburg, 138 in Durban, 82 in Cape Town and 78 in Pretoria. Even allowing for considerable under-reporting in the Transkei, this is a significant and telling difference.

What it tells of is the primary paradox of polio, viz that among those living in areas where hygiene, sanitation, sewerage and water supply were poorest, the incidence of polio was lowest. In South Africa, the bulk of such inhabitants were Africans dwelling not only in rural areas like the Transkei, Zululand and the northern, western and eastern Transvaal, but also in urban locations and slums. In polio incidence terms, the consequences were striking: in the epidemics of the 1940s, for instance, cases of paralytic polio among Africans were ten times less frequent than among whites, while in 1957 the medical officer of health (MOH) of Pietermaritzburg described the polio incidence in that city – 6/100,000 among Africans and 46/100,000 among whites – as 'the normal pattern of the disease in South Africa'.[7]

Even just among whites, this difference in incidence between those areas with good sanitary facilities and those without was noticeable: in middle-class suburbs the incidence far outstripped that in working-class areas. In Johannesburg in 1918, for example, only three of the city's 181 reported cases were from working-class suburbs.

The explanation for this paradox – which was a global phenomenon and which directly challenged the usual connection that biomedicine had been making since the 19th century between dirt and disease –

probably lies in the permanent, endemic presence of at least one strain of polio in South Africa. This meant that many children in poorly provided and insanitary areas were regularly exposed to poliovirus-contaminated food and water and, knowing little of hygiene, contracted the silent or the abortive form of the disease and thereby gained immunity. It was only if something shielded children from such early-life infection by the virus that they were left vulnerable to subsequent, newly arriving epidemics. This 'something' was the escalating roll-out of public health reforms which began in South Africa's cities early in the 20th century. As in Europe, North America, Australia and New Zealand, the first children to benefit from these reforms were the offspring of the urban middle class. In South Africa, most of these were white. With no little astonishment, South Africa's leading polio researcher concluded in 1958 that most Africans had 'acquired antibodies to all three types of poliovirus by the time they are six years old … [while] Europeans have a lower level of immunity in every age group than the corresponding age group of African[s]'.[8]

Unusually, therefore, privilege seems to have brought with it a heightened risk of polio, prompting one historian to describe this counter-intuitive situation as 'an unintended byproduct of improved sanitation … the inadvertent creation of a virgin soil population for the poliomyelitis virus … [by] sanitary regimens … [which] preserved far more infants, but left them more vulnerable to later poliomyelitis infections'.[9] The Director of the South African Institute of Medical Research labelled it, in frustration, 'the most perverse of all infective diseases'.[10]

That this anomaly was largely a function of the presence or absence of good sanitation, purified water and hygienic practices is supported by the sudden outbreak of polio on a large scale among African under-fives in East London's East Bank Location in 1956. 'The epidemic introduced a new pattern in the disease in South Africa,' commented the local MOH, 'for never before had there been an outbreak which commenced amongst Natives and was overwhelmingly confined to them.'[11] The explanation offered for this break with past trends was the recent installation of water-borne sewerage and a purified water-supply in the location, which had made the very young there less vulnerable to 'dirt' diseases but had simultaneously denied them immunity from polio. If effective prophylaxis had not very soon after this become available in South Africa, the sanitary and political implications of such an argument could have been profound.

However, none of this was known until the 1950s. Until then, the characteristics and serotypes of the virus, the forms and epidemiology of the disease, and its mode of transmission were guesswork. It is 'almost fairy-like in the mode and character of its spread … [flying] from case to case by almost untraceable channels,' declared a senior Johannesburg doctor in 1918,[12] a statement whose echo could still be heard in *The Star*'s depiction of polio 26 years later as 'a malevolent evil lurking somewhere in our midst'.[13]

Given this poor understanding of the disease, medical opinion as to how it was spread ranged from personal contact, coughing and ingesting food or drink contaminated by infected people or flies, to being bitten by virus-carrying fleas or bugs. Official advice on prevention was, accordingly, as diverse and uncoordinated. No clear lead or plan was offered by the national Department of Public Health until the 1950s, other than insisting on the need for new cases to be notified and spreading the latest knowledge about polio. For the rest, local authorities bore the brunt of combating the disease by methods chosen by their own MOHs. Consequently, their recommendations spanned a wide spectrum, from intensifying hygiene, avoiding crowds and swimming baths, and discouraging tonsillectomies to cancelling children's parties, boiling all milk, peeling vegetables and fruit, and conducting an almost frenzied war on flies. Wryly, the *South African Medical Journal* queried the last of these, as it seemed to assume that flies flew in only one direction, 'from the slums to the suburbs'.[14]

Equally common were bans on energy-sapping children's games and school sports, out of the conviction that, as a textbook on public health put it in 1959, 'sudden fatigue during competitive sport … may change the harmless infection into the paralytic disease'.[15]

To these fairly standard measures (by international standards) against polio before 1950, South Africa added a few variants, reflecting the knee-jerk racist assumptions of its authorities. Thus, ignoring the fact that relatively few cases had occurred among Africans, in 1918 African laundrymen were put under particular scrutiny by the health authorities in Johannesburg to ensure that their white clients' washing was not infected, while in 1944 the South African Railways barred African nursemaids from sitting in railway compartments with their white charges lest they convey polio to their white fellow-travellers. As always, the fear engendered by an epidemic revealed underlying notions of self and others.

If attempts at prevention until the 1950s were eclectic and unsystematic, much the same can be said of attempts at treatment of paralytic polio. Until the epidemics of the 1940s, rigid and prolonged immobilisation of the affected limbs was the norm, with splints and plaster casts widely used. By the early 1950s, however, the pendulum was swinging in the opposite direction, towards the mobilisation of withered limbs as the treatment of choice, by hydrotherapy, electrotherapy, heat therapy and physiotherapy, 'my lifeline between helplessness and mobility', as a convalescing patient called the last.[16] 'You have to learn to open the communication lines again [between nerve cells and muscles],' her physiotherapist explained. 'It will take all your patience, because you will have to go on, month after month, concentrating on each muscle in turn … But there is no other way.'[17]

Once this treatment had achieved as much rehabilitation as it could, many 'polios' (as such patients dubbed themselves) still required callipers or crutches for independent movement. In the public mind, these became the pitiful badges of polio.

Against the effects of the most dangerous form of paralytic polio in an epidemic – that which paralysed respiratory muscles – another mechanical device was, quite literally, a lifesaver. Invented in the United States in 1929, the iron lung kept hundreds of polio-paralysed patients breathing during the South African epidemics of the 1940s and 1950s. Indeed, imported iron lungs had to be supplemented by jerry-built local ones in 1944, so great was the demand. Though many patients found them claustrophobic, they were in fact the difference between life and death for them,

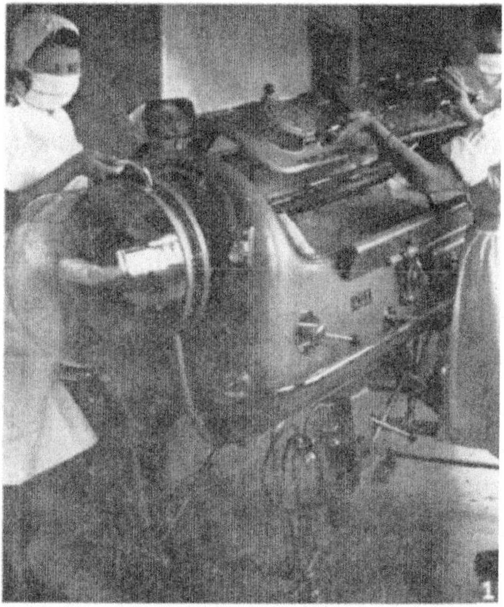

An iron lung containing an infant with polio at the Boksburg-Benoni Hospital in 1956. A reflection of the infant's unhappy face can just be seen in the mirror on top of the machine. (South African Medical Journal, *10 November 1956)*

creating an enabling space in which they could breathe with less difficulty. 'The metal respirator assumed an almost animate personality and became a symbol of protection and security,' recounted an American user of one. 'The idea of leaving it would always make our hearts beat a little faster and bring an anxious lump into our throats. We were incomplete embryos in a metal womb.'[18]

From the mid-1950s, however, the need for such

life-support machines – and indeed of all ameliorative aids – decreased, largely overtaken by the consequences of the momentous breakthroughs between 1954 and 1958, the development of effective prophylactic anti-polio vaccines.

Efforts to create such a vaccine began in the United States and South Africa after World War II, during which significant advances had been made in vaccine therapy generally. In 1948, amidst the panic of the third polio epidemic in South Africa – which saw some schools closed, others poorly attended as parents kept their children at home, baby shows cancelled, the Transvaal Dutch Reformed Church hold a day of intercession for polio victims, and even an insurance firm offering a special policy against infantile paralysis – a public appeal was launched in Johannesburg to set up a Polio Research Foundation to allow local researchers to investigate the disease thoroughly and come up with a vaccine against it. It is a mark of how deep was the fear of the disease in white middle-class homes that the response from them was enormous, despite the doubts of several prominent doctors and health officials about giving polio such priority when diseases like tuberculosis posed a much greater national threat. Middle-class volunteers went to fundraising work with a will, for instance organising a publicity-making 'Snowball Procession' across the

Witwatersrand and a children's 'March of the Tickeys' to collect funds (both in imitation of spectacularly successful initiatives of this sort by the National Foundation for Infantile Paralysis in the United States) and arranging fundraising recitals, competitions, horse shows and boxing matches countrywide. As in the United States, publicity was at the heart of the campaign, which utilised popular advertising methods utterly foreign to medical research in South Africa until then, more akin to Madison Avenue in New York than Hospital Hill in Johannesburg.

But they worked. By the end of 1949 £500,000 had been raised – almost equal to 15 per cent of the Department of Public Health's total expenditure in that year – which was used to set up the Polio Research Foundation (PRF) under the aegis of the South African Institute of Medical Research in Johannesburg. By 1953 it had built new, state-of-the-art laboratories for itself, nicknamed the 'Polio Palace', and was far advanced in developing a prophylactic vaccine. Like Jonas Salk's inactivated polio vaccine,[19] by 1954 the PRF's vaccine was ready to be piloted, making South Africa one of only four countries in the world to develop its own vaccine. However, the distribution of this vaccine was held back until September 1955 because of the need to repeat safety-checks after a batch of the Salk vaccine manufactured in California had been withdrawn when a number of children vaccinated with it in the United States had developed paralytic polio.

Despite serious reservations by some South African doctors about the PRF vaccine, its long-term effects and the duration of the immunity it promised, public demand for it rapidly outstripped the initial supply, and its roll-out had to be halted for want of vaccine until 1956, when more would be manufactured. In that year, an upsurge in polio cases, as a fourth epidemic began to emerge, quickly drained the new supply too, creating alarm and outrage among parents and, supposedly, a black market for the vaccine on the Witwatersrand. Whether it was 'one or 1000 unfortunate children and adults' who had to 'suffer as a result of inefficiency and procrastination', wrote an indignant parent, 'the guilt for the pain and misery caused to the sufferers and their relatives must fall unequivocally on those who [are] in charge of the polio [vaccine] distribution'.[20]

As the fourth epidemic intensified early in 1957, amid what one medical MP called 'great mass hysteria'[21] – which even saw a blanket ban imposed on school rugby matches – so the Department of Public Health eased its proud nationalist stance that South Africa should meet its own vaccine needs, and arranged for batches of the Salk vaccine to be imported from the United States. The pressure from up-in-arms white parents had proved too strong for the government to resist. Typical had been a hard-hitting letter from one father, declaring that 'every mother and father of a maimed, suffering or dead child will curse those responsible if the suffering is due to lack of initiative, consideration of dollars or national pride or red tape'.[22]

As a result of the government's altered stance, by 1959 all the country's vaccine needs had been finally satisfied and some 750,000 children had been vaccinated, though not without a hitch or two. The MOH of Cape Town reported in 1959 that 'Reactions to the poliomyelitis injections were minimal. Among the 98,000 injections given, the only reactions occurring were in two school children, who fainted shortly after the injection but revived rapidly after the injection of adrenalin.'[23]

Yet, as the opening paragraph of this chapter makes clear, there was an important sequel to the vaccination-by-injection campaign in South Africa. The 1956/7 epidemic had revealed that Salk's inactivated polio vaccine did not provide 100 per cent immunity and so the PRF began experimenting with making an oral polio vaccine with a weakened or attenuated poliovirus which used strains developed by another American virologist, Albert Sabin.[24]

By 1960 the PRF was manufacturing its own Sabin-type oral polio vaccine, which had the virtue of conferring immunity against all three serotypes of poliovirus with one swallow. Over the next 12 months, as free immunisation with this oral vaccine was provided nationwide, one such swallow did indeed make the summer for 5.84 million South Africans, as, for the first time in four years, they could swim and bathe without fear of contracting the 'summer virus'.

In 1963 vaccination with the oral vaccine was made compulsory for all newborns in South Africa. But by then, with notified cases having fallen to 342 per year (i.e. 10 per cent of the 1956 figure), polio epidemics were becoming a subject for historians. 'Poliomyelitis has ceased to be a major medical and research problem,' concluded the historian of the South African Institute of Medical Research triumphantly.[25]

Only for guilt-ridden parents left with crippled children and those children themselves, balancing on their crutches, callipers and canes, was it not history but their present and the future. As one of them wistfully observed about the soft metallic click as the kneelocks of his callipers engaged, 'It was a sound that governed my life.'[26]

5

HIV/AIDS, 1982–

'A catastrophe in slow motion'

'The country is busy burying its young'
– Superintendent of Hlabisa Hospital[1]

In two fundamental ways HIV/AIDS differs from the deadly epidemics already dealt with in this book. Firstly, as I write this in November 2011, it is still under way, quietly claiming over 500 lives per day. This means that this chapter lacks the historical perspective of its predecessors or even the knowledge of when and how the epidemic terminated, if indeed it ever does. Secondly, as the subtitle of the chapter indicates, HIV/AIDS is a slow-moving epidemic, for it takes at least six years for symptoms of HIV infection to manifest themselves, usually in the form of diminished resistance to other diseases, and then another one to two years for it to become terminal as AIDS. Thus it is an epidemic very different in form from those already examined, not only because of its gradual evolution and the opportunities this offers, even as it rages, to investigate it closely and develop drugs and strategies to arrest it, but also because, at the other end of the scale, those without access to such medication take several years to die, placing a lengthy demand on individuals and institutions caring for them.

Therefore, although HIV/AIDS does not possess the whirlwind-like features of its predecessors – sudden onset, explosive decimation of the population, and an intense but short-lived presence – its overall impact has, cumulatively, been no less lethal or widespread: it has claimed, directly or indirectly, some 3.3 million lives in South Africa in the 29 years since it was first diagnosed here in 1982. It may not be a *driedagsiekte* like Spanish flu, but it does not bear graphic colloquial labels for nothing, for example the two Xhosa tags, *ugawulayo* ('the chopper') and *unyathele icable* ('stepping on a live wire'). Tellingly, to some of an older generation it is 'the big flu'.

The pathogen and its course

The fact that infection with the human immunodeficiency virus (HIV) occurs primarily during heterosexual or homosexual intercourse – when an infected person's semen or vaginal secretions containing the virus are transferred into an uninfected person's system – goes a long way to explain the disease's high prevalence in South Africa's population, especially among its sexually active teenagers and young adults. In addition to them, three other groups have been at high risk of infection, viz babies born to HIV+ mothers, who might have been infected in the womb, during delivery or through taking breastmilk; haemophiliacs and transfusion recipients unwittingly receiving HIV-infected blood; and health workers who accidentally came into contact with an infected patient's blood, most commonly through a needlestick injury.

Once in a newly infected person's bloodstream, the HI virus gradually erodes the body's ability to resist other pathogens by destroying the CD4 cells at the core of the body's immune system. When an infected person's CD4 count drops from the usual 1200 cells per microlitre of blood to 200, his or her immune system is so compromised as to be unable to withstand even quite mild opportunistic, secondary infections. At this point HIV turns into full-blown AIDS from which there is no recovery unless antiretroviral drugs, which check the proliferation of the HI virus, are hastily administered. If they are not, death follows within 12 to 24 months, usually from an opportunistic disease like TB or, less commonly, from pneumonia, influenza or meningitis. HIV/AIDS and TB are therefore synergistic, HIV boosting the incidence of TB so that they in effect constitute two intertwined epidemics that complement each other. At present there is no medical cure or preventive for HIV/AIDS.

The epidemic and its course

Two subtypes or clades of the HI virus first reached South Africa in the late 1970s, along two distinct pathways. From the United States, where it had begun to manifest itself among gay men at that time, Clade B was probably introduced by one or more gay men. Two SAA air stewards who died in Pretoria in 1982 of a pneumonia that their deficient immune systems could not fight off were the first cases to be recorded in the country. Within a year, 32 more gay men in Johannesburg were diagnosed as being HIV+. Yet, this did not concern medical officials unduly, for, in their blinkered naïveté, many believed their cities to be as safe from the disease as was, supposedly, Cape Town, whose MOH expressed the opinion that 'the disease only occurred amongst homosexuals and … there were not many of those kind of people in Cape Town'.[2]

The second subtype of HIV, Clade C, appears to have been brought to South Africa a little later, from the heartland of the disease, Central and East Africa, as the first recorded cases of this clade were diagnosed among migrant Malawian mineworkers on the Witwatersrand in 1986. By then the disease was already firmly established in their homeland, Malawi, and its neighbours, and positively rampant further north in Uganda and Zaïre. Defensively, the South African Chamber of Mines was quick to point out how 'much lower than the prevalence in their home countries' was the prevalence among the Malawian miners on the Rand and that living conditions in single sex hostels there '[have] not contributed to the spread of the disease'.[3] Yet, within two months, two local women who had consorted with the Malawians were diagnosed as HIV+.

This first phase of the epidemic in South Africa, from 1982 to 1986, might thus usefully be described in meteorological terms as a pre-frontal trough which precedes a gathering storm: a handful of cases and the hope that what followed would pass quickly, without causing major damage. Keeping with the meteorological metaphor, the second phase of the epidemic, from 1986 to 1995, can be seen as the louring sky ahead of a storm, in which HIV began to spread beyond the pockets of gay men and miners and unobtrusively infect the population at large. In 1991 the number of HIV+ heterosexuals exceeded that of homosexuals for the first time, a difference which thereafter grew wider and wider as many gay men adopted safer sexual practices. By 1992 at least 2.2 per cent of pregnant women attending public-sector health facilities were HIV+, but the number of AIDS deaths still trailed far behind because of the time-lag between infection with the HI virus and escalation to AIDS. Out of a public eye at that time so focused on South Africa's watershed political transition, seeds for a generalised epidemic were being rapidly and abundantly sown.

Only once the number of AIDS deaths topped 5000 per year in 1995 – by when 10.4 per cent of pregnant women tested positive for HIV – did the threatening storm break into the open and unleash an escalating surge of morbidity and mortality, which has still not abated. This was the epidemic's third phase in South Africa, the deluge. From the mid-1990s more hearses began to be seen in rural villages at weekends and HIV support organisations like the Catholic Church's Sinosizo Project in Durban and the Buddhist Dharmagira Outreach Programme in deep rural KwaZulu-Natal were being set up in response to the burgeoning epidemic. Little wonder that health workers, confronted by a rising tide of deaths about which they could do very little, became demoralised. 'We are here to cure but now with this epidemic we are here to manage it ... We feel powerless because we don't have something to give them,' lamented one doctor in despair in 2001.[4] A nurse echoed this sentiment, insisting, 'We are like any human being faced with dying people that you can not help, it's frustrating.'[5]

By 2010, 30.2 per cent of pregnant women attending public healthcare facilities were HIV+ and AIDS deaths stood at just under 190,000 for the year. These grim features characterised the third phase of the epidemic from 1995 to date, which has made South Africa into the centre of the world's HIV/AIDS pandemic. Having been synonymous with apartheid for over 40 years, the country now became notorious for HIV/AIDS. In 2011 it contained more HIV+ people (5.6 million or 11 per cent of its entire population) than any other country in the world, while in its worst-hit provinces, KwaZulu-Natal, Mpumalanga, Free State and North-West, more than a third of pregnant women attending public healthcare facilities are HIV+.

Why did an outbreak become an epidemic?

The short answer to this fundamental question is that, like all diseases which become epidemic, HIV/AIDS rooted itself in South Africa by taking full advantage of existing social, economic, cultural and political conditions in the society. It was, in Shula Marks's apt phrase, 'an epidemic waiting to happen'[6] in perfect storm conditions. The century-old migrant labour system, which removed young African men from their rural families and concentrated them for months at a time in single-sex compounds and hostels in far-away cities, created congenial circumstances for multiple concurrent sexual relationships and thereby a high risk of contracting HIV; this was often then introduced into rural communities on the migrant's return home. In such circumstances, the existing high incidence of sexually transmitted infections (STIs) in the population and the low status of young women in patriarchal African communities made them particularly vulnerable to being infected with HIV.

Another longstanding category of men-on-the-move who expanded HIV's reach was long-distance truck drivers, who, already in the 1980s, as South Africa's road freight sector grew, were known to frequent sex-stopovers as they travelled along the country's roads and beyond its borders. Commercial sex of this sort offered many an opportunity for the HI virus to infect them and for them in turn to infect other sex workers, their wives or partners back home. In 2001, 56 per cent of sex workers tested at these stopovers were HIV+, while, of 320 truckers sampled, just over half were found to be HIV+. Among those aged 55–59, 69 per cent were HIV+. Indeed, more generally, inter-generational sex between have-men and have-not young girls (sometimes referred to as 'sex for favours') was not uncommon in late-20th-century, rapidly urbanising South Africa, with its high levels of poverty, unemployment and inequality.

This may also explain why, until antiretroviral drug therapy was publicly rolled out after 2003, those dying included a significant number of older men in regular employment. Being salaried had clearly been no bar to risky sexual behaviour. For instance, by 2000 at least ten schoolteachers were dying of AIDS-related diseases every month, while Nkandla Hospital in KwaZulu Natal lost 7 per cent and 10 per cent of its staff to AIDS in two successive years, 2004 and 2005.

At the other end of the age spectrum, the African-led youth revolt against apartheid from 1976 to 1994 also loosened traditional constraints on sexual activity in many families, as the Soweto generation rejected or ignored the conservative sexual mores of their elders in the heat of the struggle. 'It's a case of eat, drink and be merry, for tomorrow we die!' one such activist told a shocked health official who asked him in 1990 about the risk of his contracting an STI.[7] In this environment and in view of the reluctance of parents of this generation to talk about sexual matters with their children, the age of sexual debut fell sharply, to as low as 16 among half of the African teenagers surveyed in that decade.[8]

Nor did the end of apartheid alter these attitudes much. After 1994 the new democratic government in South Africa did not set about rebuilding family structures or do much to dilute the surging emphasis on sex in the media and advertising. A survey in 2000 found that one-third of boys believed that 'having many sexual partners means I am cool or hip'.[9] To many adolescent Africans in townships, to become an *isoka* ('a macho playboy') was a goal to be keenly pursued.

Apart from encouraging the development of this ethos, the end of apartheid almost certainly added to the pool of HIV+ people in South Africa from another direction, by making it possible for thousands of political exiles to return home from countries where the epidemic had been under way for over a decade. From these and other HIV-struck countries in Africa, there was also an inflow of refugees after 1994. It would be surprising if a number of these new arrivals were not HIV+.

Among African males of all ages and nationalities the risk of HIV infection was heightened by the abiding reluctance of many to use condoms, either because, before 1994, some saw using them as an apartheid-inspired ploy to curb African population growth or because a dominant culture of machismo required 'flesh to flesh' sexual intercourse. This was perceived as the only truly manly way 'of meeting male sexual desires, with condoms being seen as cold and unpleasant'. Using a condom was understood as 'wasting one's sperm' in a context where fathering many children was perceived as 'a positive sign of virile masculinity'.[10] Thus, sex workers who insisted on their use were often rejected or paid less, while in extreme cases they were beaten up by frustrated would-be clients.

On changing these entrenched sexual attitudes and practices, which together constituted what has been called the AIDS 'superhighway',[11] the apartheid government was unable to make much headway, for any steps it took were *ipso facto* deemed unacceptable by most Africans. Indeed, young militants doubted the very existence of AIDS, dismissing it as a government plot and pillorying AIDS as an '*A*frikaner *I*nvention to *D*eprive us of *S*ex'.[12] Nor was the post-1994 ANC government much more successful in altering sexual behaviour in its first dozen years in office, because of a lack of direction, capacity, co-ordination or will, especially during Thabo Mbeki's presidency (1999–2008). Tellingly, in these years a large portion of the national AIDS budget consistently remained unspent. As a result, the list of major drivers of HIV in the 2010 *South African Health Review* closely resembles the list in that review's first number 15 years earlier. As one scholar observed perceptively a decade ago, 'Vulnerability to HIV is … deeply entrenched in our social fabric.'[13]

Responses: official, unofficial, communal, individual

The official responses to the epidemic of the post-1994 national government – its apartheid predecessor's schemes were largely ad hoc and narrow in nature because of its own prejudices and the epidemic's immaturity – were embodied in six strategic or action plans tabled between 1994 and 2011. Drawing upon international best practice as recommended by the WHO and UNAIDS, the plans sought to pull in many government departments, but under the leadership of the national Department of Health. They emphasised four main terrains or platforms for action, viz prevention, treatment and care, research and human rights. What follows will examine the government's response in terms of these four platforms.

As the previous-but-one paragraph makes clear, prevention by altering sexual behaviour through exhortation, education and publicity met with very little success, despite the millions spent on it. Public awareness campaigns, the widespread preaching of the gospel of ABC ('Abstain, Be Faithful, Condomise'), the mass distribution of condoms and information brochures, the staging of a specially commissioned, AIDS-themed musical, *Sarafina 2*, and the introduction of Lifeskills as a compulsory school subject which specifically included sex education, all had but a limited impact on practice. Indeed, just talking

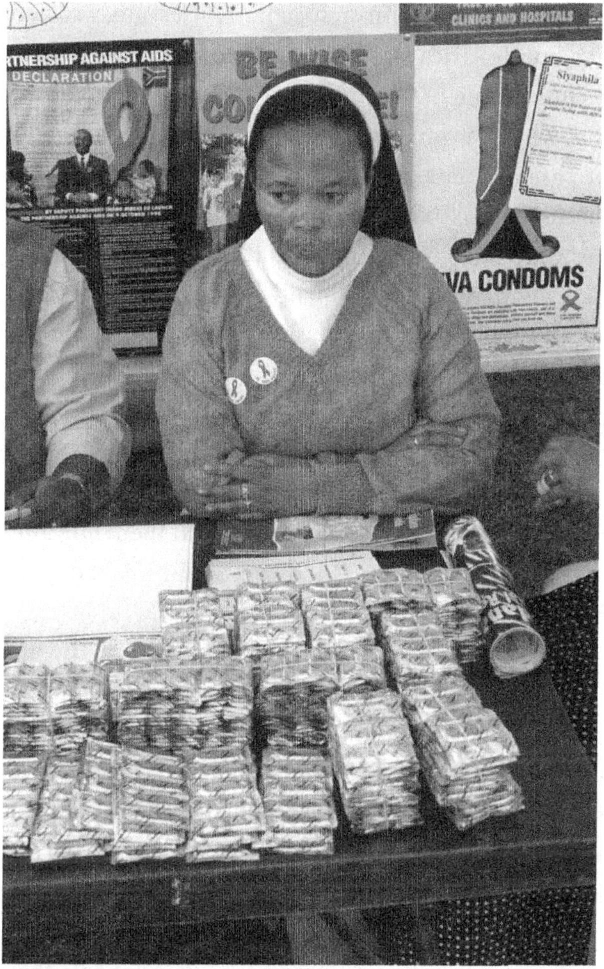

Contradictions in the midst of a crisis. A Catholic nun running a stall providing condoms in Pietermaritzburg in 2001. Officially, at this time the Catholic Church in South Africa was opposed to the use of condoms to prevent HIV infection. (Courtesy of Greg Marinovich)

about such issues in a socially conservative society like South Africa was often unwelcome. For example, a clinic sister in Mpumalanga was dismayed to find that when she taught about HIV in local schools, 'a lot of parents come to us and they complain that we are discussing sexual issues with their children and they say they don't want their children to discuss sexual issues with anybody'.[14] Equally delicate was the official adoption of male circumcision as a means to prevent the transmission of HIV, for among the Zulu this practice had been halted by King Shaka in the 1810s. Not until 2009 was the state confident enough of its preventive value to make circumcision formally part of its HIV prevention programme, and then only after the present Zulu king, Goodwill Zwelithini, had given his backing to this.

More effective were the measures taken by the central government to tackle the other modes of HIV transmission in South Africa. To reduce needlestick injuries latex gloves became standard issue for all health workers who handled patients, while protocols were amended in hospitals and clinics to curtail the use of needles where possible. To lessen the chances of infection through blood transfusions, blood banks, under governmental pressure, abandoned their practice of refusing the blood of Africans whom they judged as at high risk of being HIV+ and instead introduced more technically rigorous, HIV-sensitive screening of all donations.

The greatest official contribution to HIV prevention was the eventual provision of antiretroviral (ARV) drugs at state clinics and hospitals to prevent mother-to-child-transmission (PMTCT). Though it took nearly five years, two court cases and sustained pressure from AIDS activists and doctors to force the less-than-willing Department of Health to agree to do so in 2002, by 2006 the ARV drug Nevirapine was being offered to pregnant HIV+ women at 2525 sites around the country. The government's stated misgivings about running an extensive PMTCT programme on grounds of its high cost, infrastructural limitations and the likely toxicity and side-effects of Nevirapine were soon eclipsed by the long-term benefits of reducing the number of HIV+ newborns, from 30 per cent of all births in 2001 to 3.6 per cent in 2010.

But if foot-dragging, excuses and delays characterised official post-1994 policy on PMTCT, to the idea of treating HIV+ people with ARVs at public expense the central government was for a long time actively hostile, again for a combination of administrative, financial, infrastructural, technical and ideological reasons, the last stemming particularly from President Mbeki's denialist beliefs about the very nature and source of AIDS.

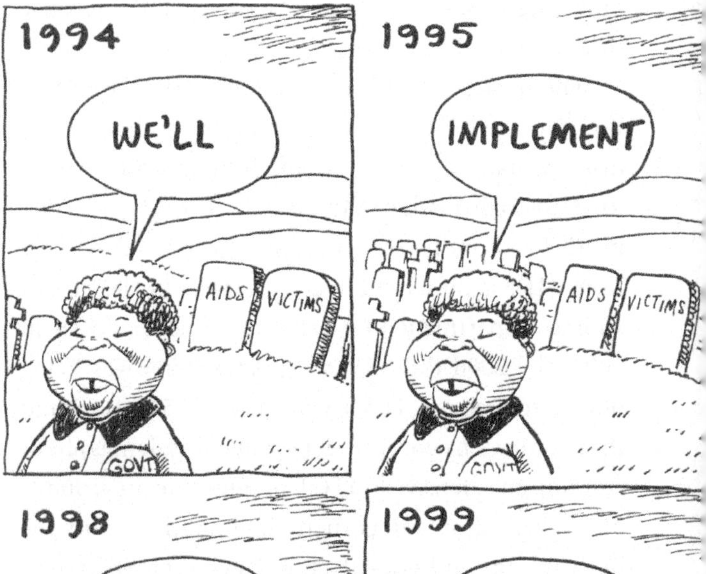

Zapiro's 2001 comment on the protracted rollout of ARVs in South Africa. The two ministers of health are Dr Nkosazana Dlamini-Zuma and her successor, Dr Manto Tshabalala-Msimang. (Cartoon by Zapiro, Sowetan *© 2001. Reprinted with permission)*

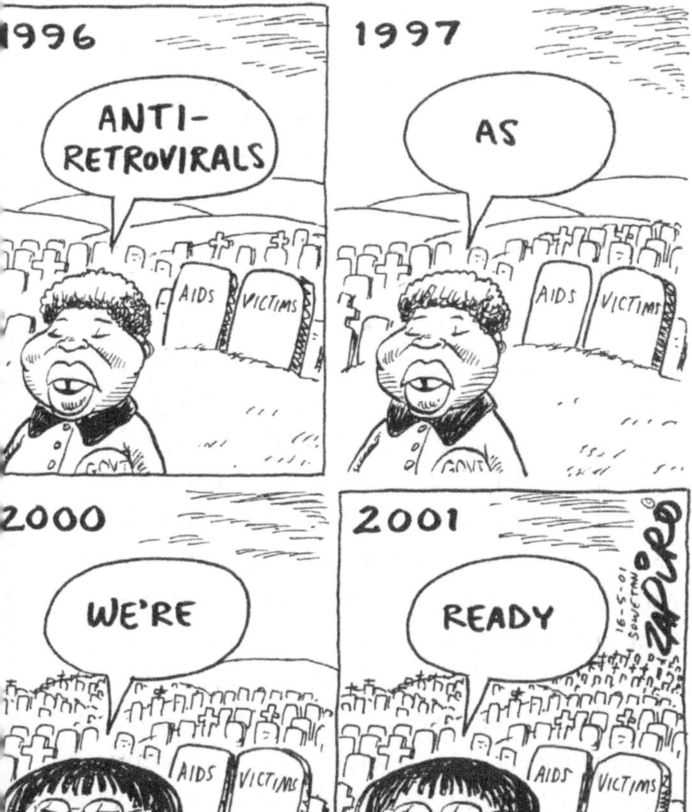
1996
ANTI-RETROVIRALS
AIDS
VICTIMS
GOVT
1997
AS
AIDS
VICTIMS
GOVT
2000
WE'RE
AIDS
VICTIMS
GOVT
2001
READY
AIDS
VICTIMS
GOVT
ZAPIRO ©
16-5-01
SOWETAN

ARV drugs – which transformed HIV from a death sentence to a chronic condition that could be managed by systematic treatment – became affordable to the public sector in South Africa in 2001, thanks to grants from international bodies like the WHO and the Global Fund Against HIV/AIDS, TB and Malaria. From that time until the cabinet's decision in 2003 to overrule President Mbeki and make these drugs readily available at state health facilities, the country was caught up in an acrimonious debate over the pros and cons of this medication. Charges that those in favour of an effective combination of three ARVs (called Highly Active Antiretroviral Treatment, or HAART) were the pawns of the big international pharmaceutical companies were traded with those by AIDS activists, who decried the people opposing them as obscurantist AIDS denialists and worse.

Yet, even after the cabinet's decision was announced, to the plaudits of AIDS activists who rejoiced that it 'changed the entire landscape of ARVT [antiretroviral therapy] in South Africa',[15] Mbeki's obdurate Minister of Health, Manto Tshabalala-Msimang – probably with his encouragement – took her time to implement the roll-out process nationally. By 2006 only some 17.3 per cent of the country's HIV+ population was receiving ARVT at public health institutions, even though the counselling and testing facilities needed for this beforehand were widely available. Exasperated, AIDS activists laid a charge of culpable homicide against her and a fellow minister who were responsible, they insisted, for the death of 600 people per day, who could have lived if they had had ARVT.

Mbeki and Tshabalala-Msimang were far keener on the roll-out of care to HIV+ people, either in the form of food supplements to keep up their health or in encouraging home- and community-based care to ease the pressure on hospitals and their staff. In her misconceived nationalist hostility to international pharmaceutical companies, Tshabalala-Msimang took her zeal even further by throwing her weight behind beetroot, garlic, lemons and African potatoes to replace ARVs as treatment for HIV/AIDS. 'We have a constitution which says people have choices to make. If people choose to use traditional medicine, why not give them those choices?' she demanded captiously.[16] Accordingly, state funds went into providing these vegetables as well as the more usual supplements, along with grants to those rendering home-based care.

More orthodox was the third component of the care programme, the energetic treatment of HIV-facilitating STIs and opportunistic infections like TB. Drawing on the country's extensive experience in combating both of these, voluntary counselling and testing (VCT) sites for HIV had TB and STI testing and treatment facilities added to what they offered, producing comprehensive Pro-Test clinics, which were gradually extended to all nine provinces.

The third terrain of the government's response to the epidemic was research. Its nationalist wish to find an African remedy to an African disease meant that it was inclined to rush in at the merest glint of a locally discovered 'magic bullet'. In 1997 it did just this, giving to two Pretoria researchers the red-carpet treatment for their supposed AIDS cure, Virodene, and pressuring the Medicines Control Council to approve it for human trials. When the Council refused, its leadership was purged amidst criticism from then Deputy President Mbeki that it was 'denying AIDS sufferers the possibility of mercy treatment to which they were morally entitled'.[17] However, the new members of the Council were equally unconvinced by the claims made for Virodene (the main ingredient of which was a highly toxic industrial solvent) and dismissed it as of 'no proven benefit for the treatment of HIV/AIDS'.[18]

Smarting at this rebuff, the government turned instead to more orthodox scientific means to combat HIV/AIDS, and in 1999 set up the South African AIDS Vaccine Initiative (SAAVI) under the eye of the Medical Research Council. The chief task of this programme was to promote and co-ordinate research to develop a vaccine to cure HIV/AIDS. With the backing of local companies and the Italian government too, the SAAVI supported several such projects, the latest one of which, the TAT Protein Vaccine, began clinical trials in 2011. Future historians of the HIV/AIDS pandemic will judge if it represents a breakthrough on a par with ARV drugs. A different project, to produce a microbicide to protect women from infection with HIV during intercourse, yielded Tenofovir gel, which is also currently undergoing trials in KwaZulu-Natal. It too will occupy either a chapter or a mere footnote in future histories of HIV/AIDS.[19]

Just as the Virodene affair made clear the ANC's political ethos, so too was this apparent in the fourth and final terrain of its AIDS policy, the safeguarding of the rights of all HIV+ people. Opposed in principle to discrimination and segregation as practised in pre-1994 South Africa, the ANC government outlawed discrimination by employers against HIV+ employees and compelled medical aid schemes to remove any restriction on the membership of those who were HIV+. Government departments were not permitted to require HIV tests of applicants for jobs, while in jails testing of prisoners was made voluntary. Moreover, those prisoners who were HIV+ were no longer allowed to be kept in separate cells from the rest of the prison population, as had been done until then.

Even the South African National Defence Force (SANDF) was forced to accept, albeit belatedly, that the HIV+ status of its members could not be a cause to exclude them from normal deployment and military duties, provided their health was up to this. 'When we are fighting or when we are doing peacekeeping work, we are not biting people. We're just being peacekeepers like anyone else,' explained one sergeant in justification. He was one of the approximately 30 per cent of SANDF soldiers who were HIV+ in 2009.[20] Unconvinced, a local defence analyst countered that this new policy introduced in 2010 was 'a massive breach of trust for ordinary soldiers … It is bad enough to [be] living under harsh conditions and running the risk of being shot at, we are now exposing them to a situation when one of their comrades could totally inadvertently infect them with a fatal disease.'[21]

Such contradictions characterised almost all of the post-1994 government's responses to the epidemic. Together they added up to a mixture of noble words and dilatory deeds, state-of-the-art advice and wrong-headed decision-making, all-inclusive schemes and perfunctory, poorly co-ordinated participation. The upshot, lamented one prominent AIDS activist in 2000, was 'grievous ineptitude', which, despite a raft of acronym-generating official task groups, workshops, committees, councils, strategic plans, action plans, proposals, statements and pledges, in fact 'signified piteously little'.[22]

For the most part, the private sector was even more behindhand in its reaction, initially averting its eyes from the looming problem or treating HIV+ employees as lepers. Only in the first decade of the 21st century did it begin to accept that HIV was, literally, business's business. Even then, as late as 2004, 75 per cent of companies surveyed lacked more than an ad hoc policy on HIV/AIDS. The 25 per cent that did have dedicated policies were usually the larger firms like Shell, Pick n Pay and Old Mutual, which had come to recognise that HIV/AIDS was affecting them increasingly through more requests for compassionate leave for employees to tend HIV/AIDS-sick relations, extended sick leave for HIV+ staff and a decline in their productivity, an accelerating loss of skills as more staff in their thirties and forties died of AIDS, and the need for greater subsidisation of medical aid membership and death benefits.

The mining industry could not, however, afford to be so tardy in its response to the epidemic. By 1992 nearly 10 per cent of just those mine employees attending STI clinics were HIV+; by 2001 some 30 per cent of all its employees were. 'There seems little doubt that the huge single-sex hostels of the gold-mining industry have become the epicenters of the

[HIV/AIDS] earthquake,' concluded a leading social economist dejectedly.[23] Negotiations with the National Union of Mineworkers (NUM) ensured that HIV+ miners would not be victimised or unilaterally fired, but the escalating magnitude of the epidemic required preventive steps too.

Early measures to prevent HIV infection among miners focused on mounting awareness campaigns, HIV testing and treatment of opportunistic infections and STIs, but their inadequacy was soon manifest. By 2001 some companies were realising that no mine is an island and began to extend their initiatives to surrounding communities where female sex workers were persuaded to become advocates of condom use and HIV education. Some mines even offered periodic STI treatment to these sex workers free of charge and were delighted when this produced a fall of 50 per cent in the incidence of STIs among their miners. This was likely to translate into a fall of 46 per cent in HIV incidence, they calculated, a saving of R2.34 million for an outlay of R268,000 for the STI treatment.

Of course, it was ultimately the compass of the bottom line by which the mining houses steered, and here projections by economists in 2000 were unequivocal: HIV/AIDS was adding R16 to the cost of producing every one ounce of gold and this might rise to R93 per ounce by 2009.

Not surprisingly, therefore, when ARV drugs became affordable in 2003, a few big mining companies like Anglo American readily made these available to their employees with a CD4 count of less than 250. As a result, such recipients of ARVT were able to work a full day, absenteeism fell by 1.9 days per employee per month, the use of in-house healthcare services declined, and so did staff turnover. Savings per patient were $93 per month in 2011. Recognising these material benefits, other mining houses followed suit; by 2006 half of the industry was providing ARVT to their employees. 'We have done the health economics and shown that for every dollar we invest in our AIDS initiatives, we get a financial return that is way in excess of that initial investment,' explained Anglo American's chief medical officer.[24]

Another reason for the mining sector's up-and-doing initiatives was pressure from its labour force through the National Union of Mineworkers [NUM]. Established in 1982, just as HIV/AIDS appeared in South Africa, the NUM was part of the country's emerging, militant black labour movement and consequently made the fight against the epidemic one of its rallying 'pillars of action', challenging the industry's actions and inaction at every turn. Indeed, within the burgeoning trade union movement as a whole, this became the norm, especially from 1985 when an overarching body, the Congress of South African Trade Unions (COSATU), was established to co-ordinate the movement. Its role was spelt out in its 'Declaration on HIV/AIDS', passed at a special congress in 1999. Noting 'the relentless advance of HIV and AIDS', this demanded 'a new approach and strategy, based on a partnership between the government and civil society in which the organised working class should play a leading role'.[25]

Of the thousand or so civil society organisations, lobby groups and survey-taking bodies that came into being after 1982 in a way not possible during shorter-lived epidemics, the Treatment Action Campaign (TAC) was the one to which COSATU gave its staunchest backing. Committed to securing treatment for those infected by HIV – many of them workers – the TAC launched itself head-on against all barriers to this goal with a missionary zeal born of the fact that many of its members were 'People Living with AIDS' (PLWA) with first-hand experience of the epidemic at grassroots level. Established in 1998 to protest against the Department of Health's decision not to roll out the provision of the early ARV drug AZT for PMTCT, it was soon going beyond this to challenge pharmaceutical companies on the high price of ARV drugs and on their opposition to the importation of generic equivalents.

In 2001 its primary target again shifted to the government, for its foot-dragging on making ARVT available nationally. Employing strategies reminiscent of the anti-apartheid struggle such as court cases, marches, petitions, media campaigns, advocacy and civil disobedience, TAC leaders like Zackie Achmat lambasted state policy, hounding and harrying responsible ministers and officials alike. Its effectiveness is evident in the breadth of the civil society coalitions it built up behind its campaigns and its achievements in changing state policy on PMTCT and ARVT. 'The TAC is the single most credible AIDS NGO in the world,' proclaimed the UN's Special Envoy on HIV/AIDS in Africa. 'It carries enormous credibility with NGOs and governments and enjoys credibility with everyone – apart from the South African government.'[26]

With its sense of purpose so positively endorsed, the TAC also sought to vanquish those who, with the tacit support of Mbeki's circle, called ARVT into question and in their place offered their own nostrums, be they vitamins, natural remedies or the miracle cures that invariably make their appearance during epidemics because of the desperate demand for an antidote at such times. Here, too, media campaigns, lobbying and court cases saw the TAC victorious. As a grassroots, single-issue, rights-based, publicity-savvy NGO, it exemplified the new social movements of the post-Cold War, post-apartheid era. Comparing it to the genteel, mass fundraising campaigns for polio research in South Africa in 1948–9 underlines the difference made by class and political culture. In effect, the polio campaign aimed at social support, the TAC at social challenge.

Social support was the thrust of many of the other NGOs active in the field of HIV/AIDS in South Africa. Their agendas were dominated by prevention through education and condom distribution, skills training to lessen poverty, voluntary counselling and testing, the promotion of home-based care and assisting AIDS orphans. Until the mid-1990s many were able to tap the not inconsiderable funding available from international donors, but thereafter much of this was channelled to the new ANC government, which was not well disposed to aiding organisations that did not toe its line. For example, between 1995 and 1998 this government cut grants to AIDS NGOs by 89 per cent. Nor was this the only direction from which the NGO sector attracted disapproval. In some communities they were perceived to be opportunistic do-gooders and know-alls who had jumped on the well-funded AIDS bandwagon. 'There is a lot of white people in NGOs and there are very few black people,' remarked a disgruntled community leader in rural KwaZulu-Natal. 'White people come in our communities with projects.

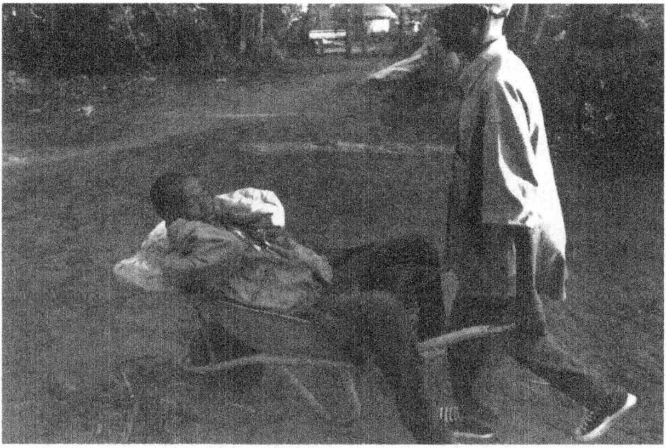

Too weak to walk by himself, a young HIV+ man from Enseleni township near Richard's Bay in KwaZulu-Natal is wheeled to an AIDS clinic by a friend in 2000. (Courtesy of Gideon Mendel)

We don't know where they get money from. They come with very little [local] help and take photos. We need NGOs that are from the community because they will have their sympathy with these people rather than a person from outside whose interest is on money.'[27]

Within such communities it was those who were HIV+ and the circle of family and friends around them, especially women, that felt the brunt of the epidemic most directly. Over the last 29 years more than 9 million of these women, men and children passed along one or more fearful paths to HIV+ status and then, if untreated, to AIDS and death. Some were steered by pluck and pressure along the 'testing–treatment' route and thereby perhaps to ongoing management of HIV as a chronic disease. Many more followed a gloomier 'symptoms–silence–cemetery' course or its tragic variant, 'disease–denial–death'. Mental and physical agony accompanied each of these journeys, along with the very human wish to make sense of why they had been infected.

As in all epidemics, whether short-lived or abiding, blaming other people for bringing a lethal infection was common and very revealing of underlying suspicions towards them. Thus, some attributed HIV/AIDS to malevolent individuals who sought every opportunity to harm them. To many Africans, human witches or wizards in the community were the most likely evil-doers as were, in the 1980s and 1990s, those whites seeking to maintain apartheid by killing off its opponents. Some even saw it as a product of Cold War germ warfare research or as an international plot by whites against blacks. For instance, in 1991 *Drum* carried without comment an article taken over from an African American journal, entitled 'Is AIDS a conspiracy against Blacks?',[28] while the ANC's house journal, *Sechaba*, claimed that 'AIDS-like viruses were being created through genetic engineering within these [US military] establishments'.[29]

On the other hand, the religious-minded saw divine punishment of sinful social or moral behaviour as the ultimate cause of the disease, especially as its chief mode of transmission was sexual intercourse. In the first phase of the epidemic, gay sex attracted particular condemnation. 'The Word of God warns against their devious form of sexuality,' thundered one Dutch Reformed Church dominee. 'AIDS proves the Biblical prescriptions. For the sake of mankind homosexual practices should be abandoned.'[30]

When the epidemic began to appear among heterosexuals too, it was their promiscuity which came under fire. One young HIV+ woman recounted in 2001 how she was rebuked by a religious doctor when she told him her status. 'He said to me I am going to die [a] terrible death. I have sinned. I have to pray to God for forgiveness because I was sleeping around. I was very angry because I did not expect that from a doctor.'[31] Not even Nelson Mandela's son, Makgatho, was spared such moral judgment. When he died of AIDS in 2004, his father was constrained to request the public not to regard the disease as 'an extraordinary thing for which people go to hell and not heaven'.[32]

Individuals' initial response to being diagnosed as HIV+ (often in a camouflaged phrase like 'There's something wrong with your blood') ranged from shock and denial to dejection and silence over their status. 'I felt that I was dead, because I told myself that OK, it was the end of the world. I will no longer live like a human being,' recalled a young man who tested HIV+.[33] For those like him who brought themselves to reveal their HIV+ status, the core support of family and friends, of members of HIV solidarity groups and of concerned nurses at ARV clinics was critical to their continued mental and physical well-being. For example, one HIV+ man remembered that 'Initially when I started she [the sister] would call me every morning at 8 a.m. to remind me [to take my medication] ... At half past 8 at night she called me [to remind me to take my second dose].'[34]

If such heartening support was not forthcoming, the prospects for coping alone were not good. Among those who committed suicide in South Africa in these years, one investigation found, HIV+ people featured disproportionately. Some families, horrified by the stigma of having an HIV+ member in their midst or terrified that they might be infected through contact, turned them out or abandoned them. As one young HIV+ woman recalled, 'My aunt used to say ... if it happens that someone in this house goes to the hospital or clinic to do an HIV test and that person is positive she will kick him or her out of the house. She chased me away after she found out.'[35] Even more extreme was the fate of people like Gugu Dlamini, a 26-year-old HIV+ woman who was beaten and stoned to death by a group of local men in KwaMashu, Durban, in 1998 for 'shaming her community' by disclosing her HIV status on television and radio programmes.

As is clear from previous chapters, stigma and blame have long been concomitants of epidemics, for nothing raises fear and an urgent need to remove its cause like the threat of death. In the case of HIV/AIDS, fear of the disease was born of a mixture of apprehension of being infected by a killer disease, ignorance about its mode of transmission and an all-too-easy identification of its source as being the sexual conduct of supposedly high-risk groups, especially if this behaviour was different from that of the mainstream. A very heterogeneous society like South Africa has never lacked for 'others' to suspect of difference; what HIV/AIDS and its predecessor epidemics added to this so powerfully was the belief that such difference could be fatal to the rest of society. In this situation, prejudice, stigma and hostility flourished and prompted action.

The extent of such stigmatisation has perhaps been diluted since 1982 by education, publicity and personal contact with PLWAs, but it still remains widespread. For instance, in 2005 more than half of the parents surveyed in Khayelitsha did not wish HIV+ staff to teach their children, while a Gauteng journalist recently noted that his HIV+ uncle had been treated by his township neighbours 'as if he was contagious, as if a handshake from him would automatically infect them ... If someone is infected the gossiping knuckleheads of the townships will discriminate or be repulsed by the sight of that person. They will either say "she was asking for it" or "shame, Z3 [a circumlocution for AIDS] is no joke, look at her now."' Angrily he concluded, 'There is so much prejudice in our black communities and families in terms of HIV/AIDS.'[36] Doctors are still often pressed by the deceased's next-of-kin not to put 'AIDS' on the death certificate as the cause of death. Indeed, in 2006 the family of a Free State woman who had died of AIDS lodged a charge of unprofessional conduct against the pathologist who had written 'AIDS' on her death certificate.

The wish to avoid incurring such prejudice and discrimination and the social disgrace that accompanied them deterred many people from being tested, for confidentiality was all too easily broken by seeing which section of a clinic people attended, how long their consultation lasted and even by what rations they received. 'When one is HIV-positive they have to eat healthy food and there is yellow maize meal that is specially made and distributed through the clinic to HIV-positive people,' explained a Limpopo man. 'We usually detect someone's HIV status by these food parcels that they carry into their home from the clinic.'[37]

For those who gave testing a wide berth, the onset of the symptoms of advanced HIV six or more years after the initial infection might be met by hiding them or attributing them to anything but AIDS. For many Africans this often led to consulting a traditional healer, but by early in the 21st century a number of such healers had been given enough information about the disease to recognise its distinctive symptoms. 'We are now aware that people sometimes have hallucinations when they are HIV-positive,' admitted a healer from rural Limpopo. 'Nowadays we don't interpret hallucinations as ancestral visitations, we refer people to the clinic to be tested for HIV when they present with hallucinations.'[38]

If they did not or could not follow the healer's advice and get onto an ARVT programme soon, the health of such patients usually deteriorated steadily as their CD4 count fell – opportunistic infections, impaired functionality, loss of appetite and weight, pain and chronic diarrhoea, which 'was the symptom that the [affected] households found most difficult to deal with', concluded a survey of such households in 2002.[39] A supportive neighbour reported of one dying PLWA, 'Leta always needs members of family to carry her from the house to the toilet. She always vomits and cry for pain and say that it can be better if she can die now. There is confusion. She acts as if she is mad and is always short-tempered.'[40]

The burden one such slowly dying patient put on

family and friends for two or more years took a heavy toll, especially as most affected families were poor. Although deprived of the sick person's income and labour, these families' financial, social and emotional resources had to cope with providing care at home and transport to a clinic or hospital. The result, as one historian put it starkly, was 'home neglect or managed death'.[41] To get a sense of the full tragedy of this in practice, it must be remembered that scenes like the following took place many thousands of times in South Africa from 1982. A mother of a dying son in Mpumalanga complained: 'He don't have a wife or children … When it looked to her like he had HIV she vanished with their three children … The hospital is too far and even if they admit him he comes back sick. His brother found him lying in bed full of sores. He coughs blood that makes it difficult to eat and we have to force him to eat or he will die … I have never benefited from this child.'[42]

In many such cases death came as welcome relief, both for the patient and the family. But in this epidemic, as in the Spanish flu two generations earlier, the death of so many young adults made it particularly tragic in character. Chief Mangosuthu Buthelezi, who lost two of his eight children to AIDS, spoke for millions of parents who had to bury a grown-up child when he confessed, 'HIV/AIDS has placed me on my knees and destroyed my family.'[43] Little wonder that today many urban cemeteries are full and that recycling existing graves and promoting cremation are high on municipal agendas. Since the onset of phase 3 of the epidemic in 1995, South Africa has become a country in a permanent state of private mourning and bereavement.

Long-term consequences

As in 1918, among those whose lives were most deeply affected by these deaths have been children who lost one or both parents to the epidemic. Nearly 2 million under-seventeens (or 11 per cent of all children) were estimated to be in this category by 2010, i.e. about five times more than a decade before, when some 2.5 per cent of all South African children were AIDS orphans.

The emotional and psychological effects of this were invariably far-reaching but are hard to measure. The social consequences are easier to describe than to assess: incorporation into the family of a relative or friend or the creation of single- or no-parent families where grandparents had to step into the breach to act as parents, often right after burying their own son or daughter. In such 'skip-generation' families the 'grandmother's burden', as AIDS has tellingly been called, could weigh heavily on the elderly. 'At my age of 59,' admitted one, 'it is hard to be a mother once again to all these children, but I try to give them all the love that I have.'[44] Where extended families could not absorb such orphans, the latter might end up living on the streets or in child-headed households. It is estimated that in 2008 nearly 100,000 children lived in such households, the bulk of them AIDS orphans. The HIV/AIDS epidemic 'has resulted in an epidemic of orphanhood and child-headed households, which has left many children having to fend for themselves', concluded an investigation into families and the youth.[45]

State intervention to ameliorate orphans' plight did not go far beyond the provision of limited social, administrative and nutritional assistance to a percentage of such child-headed households, and paying child support grants to adoptive families and orphanages. Consequently, NGOs were left with plenty of scope to innovate, for instance by setting up communal committees to place orphans with local families or by establishing 'artificial families' in which a surrogate mother was paid to care for six orphans or to lodge in the home of several related orphans and care for them. Yet, for all of these creative social innovations, the life of AIDS orphans was diminished forever. 'When AIDS takes a parent,' one scholar notes accurately, 'it usually takes a childhood as well.'[46]

The functioning of just about every family that

lost a parent to AIDS was compromised, whether in terms of its ability to nurture, to socialise, to educate, to transmit values, to discipline, to care for, to protect or to assist its members financially. To an institution which, among rural Africans at least, had already been eroded by generations of migrant labour, the HIV/AIDS epidemic added further pressure, often tipping families into dysfunctionality. And, as sociologists tell us, dysfunctional families often beget dysfunctional individual behaviour. The family and youth investigation already cited concludes that 'youth who come from dysfunctional families and communities are more likely to engage in risky behaviour and contribute to social breakdown'.[47]

Easier to measure than dysfunctionality resulting from the epidemic is its demographic impact. However, this needs to be tracked beyond just the approximately 3.3 million AIDS deaths since 1982. Not only did these deaths of predominantly young adults – deaths in the age-group 30–34 rose by 212 per cent between 1997 and 2005 – produce an uneven population pyramid, especially among Africans, who constituted a disproportionately large percentage of the dead, but they also impacted very negatively on life expectancy. Whereas in 1990 this had been 62 years, twenty years later it had dropped to 54, and that was an improvement on the figure of 51.5 in 2004, before

PMTCT and ARVT had been effectively rolled out.

The death of these young adults, HIV-induced sterility and the reluctance of some HIV+ women to bear children lest they be HIV+ too, all had an effect on births. Together with a number of socio-economic factors, they cut the annual growth of the overall population from 2.4 per cent in 1991/2 to 1.06 per cent in 2009/10. On average, the number of children conceived by each woman dropped from 2.8 to 2.5. In short, South Africa's demographic profile for the first half of the 21st century, and perhaps beyond, will bear the indelible stamp of AIDS upon it, generation by generation. One estimate calculates that the country's population would have been 77.5 million in 2040 were it not for AIDS, which will pin it back to 53.3 million.[48]

Though, in theory, ARVT has transformed the AIDS scene, in reality its ability to do so has been compromised by limited roll-out. Thus, in 2011 only 37 per cent of those eligible for ARVT are receiving such therapy, even though it is now believed that ARVT is an effective preventive measure too, as it greatly reduces an HIV+ person's infectiousness. Until this figure of 37 per cent more than doubles – the new 2012–16 National Strategic Plan aims to have 80 per cent of eligible people on ARVT within five years – attempts to check HIV/AIDS will always be playing catch-up with an epidemic whose slow-moving but inexorably lethal character (at least until ARVT is widely available) puts it into a distinctive category in South Africa's epidemic history. Yet, if its *modus operandi* is singular, the South African context in which it has blossomed is not. Like previous epidemics, the HI virus has searched out and exploited many of the same social, economic, cultural and political features which they did, and elicited many similar responses too. In that respect, HIV/AIDS is very much part and parcel of the country's 300-year pattern of epidemics. As the historian of cholera in 19th-century Russia, Roderick McGrew, observed about epidemics generally, they 'do not create abnormal situations, rather they emphasize normal aspects of abnormal situations ... An epidemic intensifies certain behavior patterns, but those patterns, instead of being aberrations, betray deeply rooted and continuing social imbalances.'[49]

6

Conclusion

As the five chapters of this book make clear, epidemics have at times been decisive in shaping South Africa's history at both the public and private level. Either as creators of new scenarios or accelerators of existing processes and trends, their significance is apparent to those who recognise the importance of disease in the making of South Africa's past.

In demographic terms, the sheer number of lives claimed and births they rendered impossible means that the shape of every South African population pyramid bears their mark. No account of the demise of Khoekhoe society or of the country's post-apartheid plight is complete without taking into consideration the epidemic factor. Moreover, to these deaths must be added their emotional, psychological and social cost to those left behind. When a history of private life, emotions and the family in South Africa comes to be written, epidemics will occur and reoccur throughout the text.

So powerful were the frightening associations that epidemics conjured up that the mere threat of one was enough to mobilise prejudices and prompt action on the public health, political or social front. Especially to South Africa's long and wretched history of forced removals and racial segregation, epidemic expediency has been a notable and, at times, critical contributor.

For biomedicine in South Africa, epidemics have usually spelled short-term defeat but longer-term success as breakthroughs like vaccination, antibiotics and antiretroviral drugs have rendered previous killer diseases preventable or at least treatable. The success of biomedicine in doing so strengthened its hand, epidemic by epidemic, over other medical systems resorted to by the population. Not the least important way in which this occurred was through the subsequent creation of official public health structures, enshrining biomedicine as the privileged, normative system of healthcare delivery.

Nor is it only as scenario-creator or process-accelerator that epidemics are important to an understanding of South Africa's past. The five chapters tellingly demonstrate that geographical mobility (especially of sailors, soldiers, impis, trekkers, truckers and migrant workers) has long been a central feature of southern African history. Even today men-on-the-move remain pivotal to the subcontinent's life and operation.

It is also clear that epidemics sharply illuminate underlying attitudes, beliefs and outlooks, religious and lay, scientific and social, medical and folk. The life-and-death situations which they create call forth raw responses and emotions unvarnished by political correctness or cosmetic politeness. Pathogens prompt prejudices with the same dire effect as epidemics elicit accusations and insinuations.

There is no way in which South Africa can escape its epidemic past. Unlike the millions of its victims, this cannot be buried. Confronting it and learning from it are what this book has sought to do.

Notes

Introduction

1 As opposed to epizootics or unusually prevalent animal diseases.

2 J. Aberth, *Plagues in World History* (Rowman & Littlefield, Lanham, 2011), 1.

3 M.W. Dols, 'The Comparative Communal Responses to the Black Death in Muslim and Christian Societies', *Viator*, 5 (1974), 275.

Chapter 1

1 D. Moodie (ed.), *The Record, or A Series of Official Papers Relative to the Condition and Treatment of the Native Tribes of South Africa* (reprint, Balkema, Cape Town and Amsterdam, 1960), 336, 386.

2 A.W. Crosby, *Ecological Imperialism: The Biological Expansion of Europe, 900–1900* (Cambridge University Press, Cambridge, 2nd edition, 2004), 197.

3 Moodie, *The Record*, 420.

4 A mild variant, *Variola minor*, first noted in the Eastern Cape in 1895, seems to have conferred a degree of immunity against smallpox on those whom it infected. Locally it was known as *amaas*, a term, linguists say, is not isiXhosa or derived from the isiXhosa word *amasi* (curdled milk). Given that by then smallpox was in retreat in the face of vaccination, the significance of *amaas* in preventing the former disease in 20th-century South Africa is uncertain.

5 Insufflation = blowing of powdered smallpox scabs up the nostrils of a recipient. Inoculation = rubbing fluid from a smallpox pustule into a cut in a recipient's skin, usually on the arm. However, among some Tswana and Pedi the cut to introduce

the fluid was made on the recipient's forehead or leg. Inoculation in this or any other form does not appear to have been carried out further south in the subcontinent, however.

6 G. Williams, *Angel of Death: The Story of Smallpox* (Palgrave Macmillan, Basingstoke, 2010), 30–1.

7 Quoted in R. Elphick, *Khoikhoi and the Founding of White South Africa* (Ravan, Johannesburg, 1985), 231–2.

8 F. Valentyn, *Description of the Cape of Good Hope, with the Matters Concerning It* (Van Riebeeck Society, Cape Town, 1971), 217, 219.

9 Quoted in R. Ross, 'Smallpox at the Cape of Good Hope in the Eighteenth Century' in C. Fyfe and D. McMasters (eds.), *African Historical Demography*, vol. 1 (Centre for African Studies, University if Edinburgh, 1977), 418.

10 H. Lichtenstein, *Travels in Southern Africa in the Years 1803, 1804, 1805 and 1806*, vol. 2 (Van Riebeeck Society, Cape Town, 1930), 287. Note that Lichtenstein used the label 'African' to refer to locally born white colonists.

11 C.P. Thunberg, *Travels at the Cape of Good Hope 1772–1775* (Van Riebeeck Society, Cape Town, 1986), 38.

12 E.H. Burrows, *A History of Medicine in South Africa up to the End of the Nineteenth Century* (Balkema, Cape Town and Amsterdam, 1958), 65.

13 S.D. Naudé and P.J. Venter (eds.), *Kaapse Plakkaatboek*, vol. 3, 1755–1783 (Cape Times, Cape Town, 1949), 17–18.

14 Valentyn, *Description of the Cape of Good Hope*, 219.

15 Naudé and Venter (eds.), *Kaapse Plakkaatboek*, vol. 3, 16.

16 R.S. Viljoen, 'Debating and Debunking Some Myths Surrounding the Decline of the Overberg Khoikhoi with Reference to the Smallpox Epidemics of 1755 and 1767' (SAHS conference paper, 1995), 12–13.

17 D.E. Stannard, 'Disease and Infertility: A New Look at the Demographic Collapse of Native Populations in the Wake of Western Contact', *Journal of American Studies*, 24 3 (1990), 337.

18 A.M.L. Robinson (ed.), *The Cape Journals of Lady Anne Barnard 1797–1798* (Van Riebeeck Society, Cape Town, 1994), 222.

19 P.C. Borcherds, *An Auto-biographical Memoir*, as quoted in E.B. van Heyningen, 'Public Health and Society in Cape Town 1880–1910' (PhD thesis, University of Cape Town, 1989), 127.

20 *South African Commercial Advertiser*, 27 October 1858, as quoted in A. Davids, '"The Revolt of the Malays": A Study of

the Reactions of the Cape Muslims to the Smallpox Epidemics of Nineteenth Century Cape Town' in C.C. Saunders, H. Phillips, E. van Heyningen and V. Bickford-Smith (eds.), *Studies in the History of Cape Town*, vol. 5 (1984), 57.

21 J. Chapman, *Travels in the Interior of South Africa*, vol. 2 (Bell & Daldy, London, 1868), 306.

22

Year	Estimated number of deaths
1713	685+
1755	2722+
1767	575+
1840	c. 3000
1858	c. 2000
1882/3	c. 4000

23 P.W. Laidler and M. Gelfand, *South Africa: Its Medical History 1652–1898* (Struik, Cape Town, 1971), 386.

24 Dr Samuel Bailey in *South African Commercial Advertiser*, 18 April 1840, as quoted in Davids, '"The Revolt of the Malays"', 63.

25 *Cape Times*, 1 August 1882, as quoted in Van Heyningen, 'Public Health and Society in Cape Town 1880–1910', 159.

26 *Cape Times*, 31 July 1882, as quoted in A. Lombaard, 'The Smallpox Epidemic of 1882 in Cape Town, with Some Reference to the Neighbouring Suburbs' (BA Honours research essay, UCT, 1981), 93.

27 Burrows, *A History of Medicine in South Africa*, 259.

28 For these accusations see respectively, Lichtenstein, *Travels in Southern Africa*, vol. 2, p. 312; P. Kirby (ed.), *The Diary of Dr Andrew Smith 1834–6*, vol. 2 (Van Riebeeck Society, Cape Town, 1940), 39; and J.B. Peires, *The House of Phalo: A History of the Xhosa People in the Days of Their Independence* (Ravan, Johannesburg, 1987), 143–4.

29 A. Offenburger, 'Smallpox and Epidemic Threat in Nineteenth-Century Xhosaland', *African Studies*, 67, 2 (August 2008).

30 J. Campbell, *Travels in South Africa* (reprint of 3rd edition, 1815, Struik, Cape Town, 1974), 4.

31 *Cape Times*, 4 September 1882, as quoted in Van Heyningen, 'Public Health and Society in Cape Town 1880–1910', 152.

32 *The Lantern*, 23 September 1882, as quoted in Davids, '"The

Revolt of the Malays'", 73.

33 Chapman, *Travels in the Interior of South Africa*, vol. 2, 300.

Chapter 2

1 S. Craddock, *City of Plagues: Disease, Poverty and Deviance in San Francisco* (University of Minnesota Press, Minneapolis, 2000), 124.

2 Cape of Good Hope, *Reports on the Public Health for 1901*, G. 66-1902, 69.

3 *Report of the Plague Advisory Board*, 1901, as cited in E.B. van Heyningen, 'Public Health and Society in Cape Town 1880–1910' (PhD thesis, University of Cape Town, 1989), 304.

4 *Report by Medical Officer of Health, Cape Town*, 1900–1, as cited in M. Swanson, 'The Sanitation Syndrome: Bubonic Plague and Urban Native Policy in the Cape Colony, 1900–1909', *Journal of African History*, 18, 3 (1977), 392.

5 *Rand Daily Mail*, 24 March 1904 (letter from V.G. Naidoo and V. Kathanpillay, on behalf of Madrassa and Colonial-born Indians).

6 Morbidity and mortality figures, 1901–7

	Cases	Deaths
Cape Town	764	371
Port Elizabeth	343	183
Durban	201	145
Johannesburg	113	82
East London	96	61
King William's Town	64	33
Rest of southern Africa	133	83
Total	1714	958

Note the high incidence in port cities but the almost entire absence of cases in inland cities like Kimberley, Bloemfontein and Pretoria. Sources for the above: Cape of Good Hope, *Report of the Medical Officer of Health for the Colony on Public Health for 1904 and 1905*, G. 39-1906, liv; E. Hill, *Report on the Plague in Natal 1902–3* (Cassell, London, Paris and Melbourne, 1904), 1; Transvaal (Colony), *Rand Plague Committee, Report upon the Outbreak of Plague on the Witwatersrand March 18th to July 31st,*

1904 (Johannesburg, 1905), 12, 15; S.E. Caldwell, 'The Course and Results of the Plague Outbreaks in King William's Town, 1900–1907' (BA Honours dissertation, Unisa, 1987), 53; E.H. Cluver, *Public Health in South Africa* (CNA, Cape Town, 1959), 197.

7 The *Yersinia pestis* bacillus had been identified as the causative pathogen of plague by two bacteriologists working independently in Hong Kong in 1894, Alexandre Yersin and Shibasaburo Kitasato, while a French bacteriologist working in Bombay, Paul-Louis Simond, had put forward the argument in 1898 that the rat flea was the vector of the disease. It took over a decade for this to be generally accepted by the medical profession.

8 Dr Gilchrist, *Rand Daily Mail*, 21 March 1904.

9 Professor W.J. Simpson, 1901, as cited in Van Heyningen, 'Public Health and Society in Cape Town', 312.

10 Dr George Turner, *The Star*, 29 March 1904.

11 Hill, *Report on the Plague in Natal*, 2–3.

12 Cited in M.W. Swanson, '"The Durban System": Roots of Urban Apartheid in Colonial Natal', *African Studies*, 35, 3–4 (1976), 168.

13 Cited in Swanson, 'The Sanitation Syndrome', 392.

14 Cited in Caldwell, 'The Course and Results of the Plague Outbreaks in King William's Town', 39.

15 Swanson, '"The Durban System"', 171; K.S.O. Beavon, 'Black Townships in South Africa: Terra Incognita for Urban Geographers', *South African Geographical Journal*, 64, 1 (1982), 8.

16 Cape of Good Hope, *Reports on the Public Health for 1901*, G. 66-1902, 93.

17 *Rand Daily Mail*, 22 March 1904; Transvaal (Colony), *Rand Plague Committee, Report*, 63.

18 Swanson, 'The Sanitation Syndrome', 387.

19 Transvaal (Colony), *Rand Plague Committee, Report*, 76.

20 *The Collected Works of Mahatma Gandhi* (Electronic Book), New Delhi, Publication Division Government of India, 1999, vol. 3, letter 309, *Indian Opinion*, 16 April 1904.

21 *Imvo Zabantsundu*, 1 March 1903, as cited in Caldwell, 'The Course and Results of the Plague Outbreaks in King William's Town', 28.

22 Dr Waldemar Haffkine, a bacteriologist trained at the Pasteur Institute, had developed a crude but effective anti-plague vaccine in 1897 while working in Bombay.

23 *Imvo Zabantsundu*, 18 June 1901, as cited in J.F. Kirk, *Making a*

Voice: African Resistance to Segregation in South Africa (Westview Press, Boulder and Oxford, 1998), 180.

24 Transvaal (Colony), *Rand Plague Committee, Report*, 82.

25 *Cape Mercury*, 17 June 1901, as cited in Caldwell, 'The Course and Results of the Plague Outbreaks in King William's Town', 13.

26 Cape of Good Hope, *Report of Medical Officer of Health for the Colony on Public Health, 1903*, G. 35-1904, 260.

27 For comparison, plague deaths in Hong Kong in 1894 were 2552 and in Bombay in 1896/7 10,760. The case mortality in these two cities was very high, 95 per cent and 83 per cent respectively (M. Echenberg, *Plague Ports: The Global Impact of Bubonic Plague 1894–1901* (New York University Press, New York and London, 2007), 314).

28 Hill, *Report on the Plague in Natal*, 3.

29 Swanson, 'The Sanitation Syndrome', 393, 396.

30 Alfred Mangena, 1901, as cited in C.C. Saunders, 'The Creation of Ndabeni: Urban Segregation and African Resistance in Cape Town' in C.C. Saunders (ed.), *Studies in the History of Cape Town*, vol. 1 (University of Cape Town, Cape Town, 1979), 150.

31 *Cape Argus*, 20 February 1901, as cited in Echenberg, *Plague Ports*, 291.

32 Saunders, 'The Creation of Ndabeni', 142.

33 *Eastern Province Herald*, 23 January 1902, as cited in A.J. Christopher, 'Race and Residence in Colonial Port Elizabeth', *South African Geographical Journal*, 69 (1987), 12.

34 *Cape Daily Telegraph*, 14 April 1905, as cited in Kirk, *Making a Voice*, 239.

35 G.F. Baines, 'The Control and Administration of Port Elizabeth's African Population, c.1834–1923', *Contree*, 26 (1989), 18.

36 Cited in Caldwell, 'The Course and Results of the Plague Outbreaks in King William's Town', 43.

37 Natal Department of Public Health minute, 1903, as cited in Swanson, '"The Durban System"', 171.

38 *The Star*, 13 October 1904.

39 *The Star*, 10 October 1904.

40 *The Star*, 13 October 1904.

Chapter 3

1 'So-called' because the only reason for the label 'Spanish' was that, unlike most countries where the epidemic struck, Spain was

not at war in 1918 and so did not censor press reports about the epidemic's presence there.

2 *Daily Dispatch*, 28 September 1918.

3 Western Cape Provincial Archives and Records Repository, Cape Town, 1/TSO 11, file 485 (1), Telegram from Magistrate Tsolo to Chief Magistrate Transkei, 16 October 1918.

4 *People's Weekly*, 12 October 1918.

5 *Daily Dispatch*, 4 November 1918.

6 *Christian Express*, 2 December 1918, 185.

7 Witwatersrand University Library, Historical and Literary Papers Division, AB 1011 (Bishop J.W. Williams Papers), Diary 1918–19, entry for 9 November 1918.

8 *The Friend*, 8 November 1918.

9 *Uitenhage Times*, 16 October 1918.

10 *Debates of the House of Assembly … as Reported in the Cape Times*, vol. 4 (1919), 51, col. 3.

11 National Archives Repository, Pretoria, Acc. 172, vol. 2, E.O. Müller, 'Lewensloop', 37–8 (translation by author).

12 Interview by author with Mr P.J. du Plessis, 20 January 1981.

13 *South African Medical Record*, 14 February 1919, 364.

14 Letter to author from Dr R.L. Forsyth, 2 November 1978.

15 Western Cape Provincial Archives and Records Repository, Cape Town, Kimberley City Council Minute Book 18, p. 55, 'Report to Mayor and City Councillors from Deputy Mayor, Cllr. C.W. Lawrence on Organisational Work to Combat Epidemic of Spanish Influenza, 7th November, 1918', 25.

16 W.H. Dawson, *South Africa: People, Places and Problems* (London, 1925), 252.

17 Library of Parliament, Cape Town, 'Union of South Africa, Commission on the Influenza Epidemic, Evidence 1918–1919', vol. 1, file 5, Evidence of A. Stewart, 1.

18 Ibid., 'Memorandum on Progress of Epidemic in Bloemfontein Submitted by J.P. Logan', entry for 14 October 1918.

19 *Cape Argus*, 14 October 1918.

20 *De Koningsbode*, July 1919, 141 (translation by author).

21 *Evening Post*, 28 August 1965.

22 *Daily Dispatch*, 21 January 1919.

23 *Cape Times*, 13 April 1920.

24 National Archives Repository, Pretoria, PM 1/1/449, file PM 1/30/10/19, Report on the Public Health Act by E.L. Mathews,

Law Adviser, 29 July 1919, 4.

25 *Die Huisgenoot*, March 1919, 676 (translation by author).

26 C.M.J. Aarts de Vries, *Ziekeverpleging in Huis* (Cape Town, 1919), preface (translation by author).

27 *Cape Times*, 16 July 1929.

28 *Cape Times*, 31 October 1919.

29 *Debates of the House of Assembly … as Reported in the Cape Times*, vol. 8 (1923), 67, col. 3.

30 Interview by author with Mrs M. Jones, 14 June 1978.

Chapter 4

1 T. Gould, *The Summer Plague* cited in M.M. Wade, '"Straws in the Wind": Early Epidemics of Poliomyelitis in Johannesburg, 1919–1945' (MA thesis, UNISA, 2006), 4.

2 Wade, ' "Straws in the Wind" ', 245.

3 The *Oxford English Dictionary* dates the first use of the term 'poliomyelitis' to 1878. The first use in print of the abridged form 'polio' dates to 1911.

4 C.J. Rutty, 'The Middle Class Plague', cited in Wade, '"Straws in the Wind"', 1.

5 Cited in Wade, '"Straws in the Wind"', 93.

6 E. Foster, *It Can't Happen to Me* (Howard Timmins, Cape Town, n.d.), 4, 15, 16–17.

7 City of Pietermaritzburg, *Report of the Medical Officer of Health for 1957*, 12.

8 J. Gear, 'The Epidemiology of Poliomyelitis in Africa', 930; www.lib.itg.be/open/ASBMT/1958/1958asbm0927.pdf.

9 J.N. Hays, *Epidemics and Pandemics: Their Impacts on Human History* (ABC Clio, Santa Barbara, 2005), 378, 414, 415.

10 E.H. Cluver, *Public Health in South Africa* (CNA, Cape Town, 1959), 238–9.

11 Municipality of East London, *Report of the Medical Officer of Health, 1945–1956*, 49.

12 Cited in Wade, '"Straws in the Wind"', 75–6.

13 *The Star*, 25 November 1944, as cited in Wade, '"Straws in the Wind"', 184.

14 *South African Medical Journal*, 25 November 1945, cited in Wade, '"Straws in the Wind"', 194.

15 Cluver, *Public Health in South Africa*, 239.

16 Foster, *It Can't Happen to Me*, 17.

17 Foster, *It Can't Happen to Me*, 20.
18 D.J. Wilson, *Living with Polio* cited in Wade, '"Straws in the Wind"', 206.
19 A team led by Jonas Salk (1914–95), a virologist at the University of Pittsburgh, had developed an effective vaccine against polio using inactivated (or dead) specimens of the poliovirus. It was administered by injection.
20 Letter in *Cape Times*, 13 November 1956, cited in W.K. Bettzieche, 'Polio, People and Apartheid: The South African Poliomyelitis Epidemics of the 1940s and 1950s with special reference to the Cape Peninsula' (BA Honours dissertation, UCT, 1998), 76.
21 Dr Carel de Wet as cited in Bettzieche, 'Polio, People and Apartheid', 78.
22 Letter from E.J. Oppenheimer in *Cape Argus*, 12 February 1957, cited in Bettzieche, 'Polio, People and Apartheid', 77.
23 Corporation of the City of Cape Town, *Annual Report of the Medical Officer of Health for 1959*, 31.
24 A team led by Albert Sabin (1906–93), a virologist at Cincinnati Children's Hospital, had developed an anti-polio vaccine using an attenuated specimen of the poliovirus. It was administered by mouth. Sabin was fiercely critical of Salk's vaccine.
25 M. Malan, *In Quest of Health: The South African Institute of Medical Research 1912–1973* (Lowry Publications, Braamfontein, 1988), 242.
26 B. Michel cited in Wade, '"Straws in the Wind"', 219.

Chapter 5

1 Superintendent of Hlabisa Hospital cited in J. Iliffe, *The African AIDS Epidemic: A History* (Ohio University Press, Athens and Double Storey, Cape Town, 2006), 45, note 55. The chapter subtitle is from Susan Sontag's *AIDS and its Metaphors* (Penguin Books, London, 1989), 88.
2 Cited in L. Grundlingh, 'HIV/AIDS in South Africa: A Case of Failed Responses Because of Stigmatization, Discrimination and Morality, 1983–1994', *New Contree*, 46 (November 1999), 63.
3 South African Chamber of Mines, *97th Annual Report*, 1986, 15.
4 *South African Health Review*, 2002, 196.
5 *South African Health Review*, 2005, 142.
6 S. Marks, 'An Epidemic Waiting to Happen? The Spread of HIV/AIDS in South Africa in Social and Historical Perspective', *African*

Studies, 61, 1 (2002), 13.

7 Quoted in V. van der Vliet, 'AIDS: Losing "The New Struggle"?', *Daedalus*, 130, 1 (Winter 2001), 159.

8 *South African Health Review*, 2003–2004, 203.

9 *South African Health Review*, 2001, 166.

10 C. Campbell, Y. Mzaidume and B. Williams, 'Gender as an Obstacle to Condom Use: HIV Prevention among Commercial Sex-Workers in a Mining Community', *Agenda*, 39 (1998), 52.

11 H. Epstein, *The Invisible Cure: Africa, the West and the Fight Against AIDS* (Farrar, Straus and Giroux, 2007), xviii

12 Van der Vliet, 'AIDS', 155.

13 South African Institute of Race Relations, *South Africa Survey*, 2001/2002, 42.

14 *South African Health Review*, 2006, 99.

15 *South African Health Review*, 2003–2004, 330.

16 South African Institute of Race Relations, *South Africa Survey*, 2006/2007, 357.

17 South African Institute of Race Relations, *South Africa Survey*, 1997/1998, 183.

18 Cited in J. Myburgh, 'The Virodene Affair, III' (18 September 2007) at http://www.politicsweb.co.za.

19 On 25 November 2011, two days after I wrote the text on page 131, trials with this gel were halted as it was found to be ineffective in preventing HIV. Tenofovir will therefore be a mere footnote. This well illustrates the pitfalls of writing history while it is still happening.

20 Cited in K. Allen, 'South African Troops Win Biggest Battle' (1 December 2009) at http://news.bbc.co.uk/2/hi/africa/8386280.stm.

21 Cited in K. Allen, 'South African Troops Win Biggest Battle' (1 December 2009) at http://news.bbc.co.uk/2/hi/africa/8386280.stm.

22 Mr Justice Edwin Cameron cited in Van der Vliet, 'AIDS', 177.

23 South African Institute of Race Relations, *South Africa Survey*, 2001/2002, 25.

24 *Mail & Guardian*, 25 November 2011, 'World Aids Day Supplement', 2.

25 Cited at http://www.cosatu.org.za/show.php?=1960.

26 South African Institute of Race Relations, *South Africa Survey*, 2006/2007, 357.

27 *South African Health Review*, 2006, 101.
28 *Drum*, February 1991, 16.
29 Mzala, 'AIDS and the Imperialist Connection', *Sechaba*, 22, 11 (November 1988), 28.
30 Cited in Grundlingh, 'HIV/AIDS in South Africa', 61.
31 *South African Health Review*, 2001, 195.
32 Cited at http://www.sahistory.org.za/dated-event/makgatho-mandela-dies.
33 *South African Health Review*, 2001, 191.
34 *South African Health Review*, 2006, 100.
35 *South African Health Review*, 2001, 191.
36 M. Manaka, 'From the Cradle to the Grave in Africa', *Mail & Guardian*, 4 November 2011.
37 *South African Health Review*, 2006, 97.
38 *South African Health Review*, 2006, 98.
39 *South African Health Review*, 2002, 203.
40 *South African Health Review*, 2002, 208.
41 Iliffe, *The African AIDS Epidemic*, 110.
42 *South African Health Review*, 2002, 210.
43 Cited at www.journaids.org/index.php/essential_information/hivaids_key_people/mangosuthu_buthelezi/
44 Cited in Iliffe, *The African AIDS Epidemic*, 118.
45 South African Institute of Race Relations, *Fast Facts*, April 2011, 7.
46 Cited in Iliffe, *The African AIDS Epidemic*, 117.
47 South African Institute of Race Relations, *Fast Facts*, April 2011, 7.
48 South African Institute of Race Relations, *South Africa Survey*, 2009/2010, 1, 5.
49 R. McGrew, 'The First Cholera Epidemic and Social History', *Bulletin of History of Medicine*, 34 (1960), 71.

Index

Achmat, Zackie 137
acquired immunity to disease 14, 16, 19, 25, 100
AIDS, *see* HIV/AIDS
Africans: blaming 71, 73; incidence of AIDS among 119–21; incidence of polio among 98; residential segregation 53, 55, 59–60, 61–7
antiretroviral (ARV) drugs and therapy 125–9, 135, 136–7, 150–1
'Black October', *see* Spanish flu
bubonic plague, *see* plague
Buthelezi, Mangosuthu 146
Cape Times Fresh Air Fund 91
cattle killing in Transkei 34
Christian responses to disease 23, 28, 34–5, 140–1
civil society organisations and HIV/AIDS 136–7
condoms and HIV/AIDS 120–1, 123
conspiracy theories 33–4, 71, 73, 121, 140
Coolie Location 44, 50, 52, 53, 54, 56, 64
COSATU (Congress of South African Trade Unions) 136
demographic impact of epidemics 25–6, 59, 82–5, 92, 149–50, 152
Dlamini, Gugu 142
epidemic expediency 51
epidemics, an overview 9–11
epidemics, and men-on-the-move 153–4
fodder imports and bubonic plague 42–3
geographical mobility and epidemics 153–4
Ginsberg Location 63
HIV/AIDS 111–51; and families 147–9; and public health 129; blame for 140–1; colloquial terms for 112; demographic impact 149–50; denialism 125; different from other epidemics 111–12; discrimination 131–2; divine punishment 141; epidemic and its course 114–17; first cases 114; from outbreak to epidemic 117–21; government response

to 122–33; individuals' response to 141–7; long-term consequences 147–51; pathogen and its course 112–14; preventive measures 124, 134; private sector response to 133–8; public health measures 124; South African National Defence Force 132; social support for communities 138–41; statistics 118, 149–50; stigmatisation 143–4; symptoms 145–6
infantile paralysis, *see* poliomyelitis
influenza, *see* Spanish flu
International Sanitary Conference (1897) 41
iron lungs 104–6
isolation, a natural preventive against disease 13, 14
Jenner, Edward 17, 26
Khoekhoen: beliefs about smallpox 23–4; burials 19, 20; effects of smallpox on 14–15, 17–19, 24–6; pre-colonisation 13–14
Klipspruit Location 53–4, 64–6
life assurance post Spanish flu 87, 93
Mandela, Makgatho 141
Mbeki, Thabo 125, 128–30
migrant labour and HIV/AIDS 117–18; and Spanish flu 70
mining sector and HIV/AIDS 115, 133–6
mother-to-child transmission of HIV/AIDS 113, 125, 136, 137
Muslims: attitudes towards 36; reaction to epidemics 23, 28, 30–2, 33–4
Ndabeni Location 60
New Brighton Location 62–3
Nevirapine 125
NGOs and HIV/AIDS 138–9
non-immune populations 18, 28
NUM (National Union of Mineworkers) 134, 135–6
Orenstein, Alexander 79
orphans 84–5, 147–9
Pinelands 91
plague 38–67; and racial prejudice 49–57; blame for 49–57; bubonic 38–9; epidemiology 42–5; first cases 41–3; history 39–43; in Cape Town 42–3, 53, 59–61; in Durban 64; in Johannesburg 44, 52, 53–4; in King William's Town 57, 63–4; in Port Elizabeth 50, 55, 61–3; inoculation programmes 57; long-term impact 66–7; medical opinions 46–9; pneumonic 39; preventive measures 48–9; social and political import 59–67; spreads in South Africa 43–6; statistics 43, 45, 58–9; symptoms 39, 45–6; vaccine 55
PMTCT (prevent mother-to-child transmission) 125, 136, 137
poliomyelitis 94–110; a middle-class disease 95–6; and public health 100–1; course of the disease 96–7; epidemiology 97–9; first cases 95; fundraising for 106–7; in Durban 98; in rural areas

98–9; on Witwatersrand 98; preventive measures 102–3; public health measures 100–1; statistics 98, 99; symptoms 97; treatments 103–10; troops a likely vector 98; vaccines and vaccination 106, 107–10
Port Elizabeth Plague Board 55
racial pathologising 51
racial segregation and the plague 59–67
railway systems and spread of infection 44, 80–1, 82
Rand Plague Committee 52, 53, 57
rats and the plague 39, 42–4, 46–8, 50, 58
religious responses: to biomedical precepts 28–32; to disease 23, 33–5, 86, 140–1
Salk vaccine 107–9
Sarafina 2 122
sex instruction and HIV/AIDS 123–4
sex workers and HIV/AIDS 118, 121, 134
sexual activity and HIV/AIDS 112–13, 119–21, 141
slaves and smallpox 19, 22, 23–4
smallpox 13–37; blame for 23–4, 33–4, 36; colloquial terms for 16; demographic impact 25–6, 59; epidemiology 13–16, 28–9; first cases 14–15; in Cape Town 17–19, 26–32; in pre-vaccination age 17–26; in vaccination age 17, 26–37; origins 15, 17–18; preventive measures 16–17, 21–4, 26–8, 29–30; public health measures 32–3, 35–6; statistics 18–19, 27, 29, 33; symptoms 15–16, 18
South African AIDS Vaccine Initiative 130–1
Spanish flu 68–93; blame for 71, 73; colloquial terms for 68, 75; corpses and burials 71, 73–4; demographic impact 82–5, 92; differential impact 81–2; epidemiology 69–71, 80–2; first cases 69; in Bloemfontein 70, 79–80; in Cape Town 70, 72, 73–4; in Cathcart district 71; in Kimberley 70, 74, 79; in Mt Frere and Mt Ayliff 82; public health afterwards 87–90; statistics 68, 70, 80–1, 82; symptoms 75–6; treatments 76–9; Union Defence Force 78–9
TAC (Treatment Action Campaign) 136–8
Tenofovir gel for HIV/AIDS 131
traditional beliefs against biomedical precepts 23, 28–32
traditional healers 77, 129, 145
travel restrictions to control disease 54–5, 103
truckers and HIV/AIDS 118
Tshabalala-Msimang, Manto, and HIV/AIDS 126, 128–9
tuberculosis (TB) 10, 113–14, 129–30
Uitvlugt Location 53, 57, 59–60
Variola major, *see* smallpox
Virodene for HIV/AIDS 130, 131
Waaihoek African township and influenza 79–80
Xhosa reaction to smallpox 21, 34
Yersinia pestis 38, 39, 46, 92